Acid Alkaline Balance: The Missing Link to Health

Dr. Susan's Healthy Living
drsusanshealthyliving.com

Facebook.com/DrSusanRichards
drsusanshealthyliving@gmail.com
(650) 561-9978

ISBN 978-1511976596

Note

The information in this book is meant to complement the advice and guidance of your physician, not replace it. It is very important that any person who has medical problems be evaluated by a physician. If you are under the care of a physician, you should discuss any major changes in your regimen with him or her. Because this is a book and not a medical consultation, keep in mind that the information presented here may not apply in your particular case. In view of individual medical requirements, new research, and government regulations, it is the responsibility of the reader to validate health practices and treatments with a physician or health service.

Table of Contents

PART 1: How Acid-Alkaline Balance Affects Health and Wellness

Introduction to Part 1

Dear Friend,

Would you like to have great health and resistance to disease, boundless energy and stamina and a positive and optimistic mood? Then, having a healthy acid-alkaline balance is essential for both your health and quality of life. I have seen the importance of having a healthy acid-alkaline balance in many thousands of patients in my clinical practice and the importance of this condition has been researched in thousands of studies.

In its natural, healthy state, the human body is slightly alkaline. Virtually all of our cells and tissues contain significant amounts of alkaline substances, such as minerals, oxygen, and bicarbonate. Our blood must maintain a state of slight alkalinity for our very survival. Almost all of our crucial bodily functions—including immunity, digestion, and cardiovascular health—as well as most of our metabolic processes and enzyme reactions require a slightly alkaline internal environment. It follows, then, that both peak performance and optimal health depend on the body's ability to maintain a slightly alkaline state in virtually all of our cells and tissues. The benefits of maintaining this healthful state of slight alkalinity are summarized in the following chart.

Most healthy individuals are readily able to maintain a healthful state of slight alkalinity, which allows them to live life to the fullest and provides them with tremendous energy and stamina. Since healthy people experience very little downtime, they epitomize Woody Allen's observation that 80 percent of success is "just showing up." They are able to persevere and meet their goals when everyone else has dropped by the wayside.

A slightly alkaline state is also necessary if one is to maintain the ability to solve complex mental problems or sustain the creativity needed to make breakthroughs in any field. It also supports our ability to socialize and create strong personal relationships. Finally, when our cells and tissues are slightly alkaline, we are better able to ward off or quickly recover from minor illnesses such as colds, flus, sinusitis, and allergies. We are also able to recover rapidly from injuries, minor surgery, and the effects of vigorous physical activity.

In contrast, when your cells and tissues are overly acidic, you tire easily and are often fatigued. It becomes more difficult to think clearly. You are more likely to develop a pessimistic outlook on life. Even if you have high goals and aspirations in life, you will lack the energy and vital spark to carry them out to their fullest extent.

Overacidity decreases your resistance to colds and flus. You are more likely to suffer from allergies that leave you bleary-eyed and tired at work or sleepy from the drugs you take to suppress the symptoms. Frequent episodes of these minor respiratory illnesses cause millions of Americans to miss work, athletic events, and social engagements.

It also contributes to conditions like arthritis, which can interfere with the ability to succeed in our information economy. It can cause your fingers to become stiff and sore so that you are unable to use a computer, or it can cause hip pain that makes it difficult to sit at a desk for any length of time. Eventually, this inability to neutralize acids in the body causes the slow movements and stiffness of the elderly and contributes to chronic, long-term medical problems like high blood pressure, autoimmune diseases, cancer, and, finally, death itself.

In my book, I share with you how to restore your body to a state of healthy acid-alkaline balance in which your cells, tissues and organ can maintain their natural, slightly alkaline state. This is a program that has benefited many thousands of my patients and has helped to restore them to optimal health and wellness. I look forward to my program providing you with similar great benefits. To accomplish this goal, I have divided the book into two parts.

Various physical traits, abilities, and health conditions can serve as helpful indicators of whether your body is fundamentally acid or alkaline. I recommend that you work through the following checklists (photocopy them if you don't want to write in the book), and refer to them as you read through the chapter. Doing so will give you a better general idea of whether your own system tends toward acidity or alkalinity.

In Part 1, I focus on how acid–alkaline balance affects health and wellness. I have included chapters on the chemistry of acid-alkaline balance and how this system functions within the body. Next, I discuss the effects of diet, lifestyle and aging have on acid alkaline balance. I then share with you how acid-alkaline balance affects many common illnesses as well as crucial peak performance traits. This will help you to understand the important role that healthy acid-alkaline balance plays in our everyday lives. Finally, I provide you with simple self-tests as well as information on laboratory tests that your doctor can order that will give you an indication of your acid-alkaline balance.

In Part 2, I share with you my very effective and powerful four-part program that will enable you to restore your body to its healthy, slightly alkaline state. You will benefit greatly from my program which includes:

1.   Following the alkaline power diet.

2.   Restoring the alkaline mineral reserves of your cells, tissues, and bones.

3.   Using alkalinizing agents for quick symptom relief.

4.   Initiating healthy lifestyle changes to reduce the stress on your buffer systems and organs of elimination.

As you begin to reduce the acid load of your body and restore your mineral reserves and buffer systems and reduce the stress on your organs of elimination, you will begin to see astonishing results in your level of performance in many crucial areas. You will also begin to experience a significant improvement in your health. Your level of physical energy, mental clarity, emotional well-being, and even optimism and creativity will be enhanced as your body regains its healthful alkalinity. The frequency of respiratory illnesses like colds, flus, and sinusitis should begin to drop dramatically. Aches and pains, heartburn, allergies, and many other chronic ailments should also begin to diminish in intensity and, finally, disappear. I look forward to you benefiting greatly from the information in this book.

Love,

Dr. Susan

Benefits of Acid-Alkaline Balance

Peak-Performance Benefits

- Increased physical vitality and stamina

- Ability to handle career and job stress

- Enhanced mental clarity and acuity

- Increased ability to get along with other people

- Increased optimism and vision

Health Benefits

- Increased resistance to illness (includes colds, flus, sinusitis, bronchitis, and pneumonia)
- Hastened recovery from illness, injury, and exertion (including colds, flus, sinusitis, bronchitis, pneumonia, allergies, and traumatic injury or surgery)
- Reduces incidence of digestive problems such as heartburn, irritable colon, Crohn's disease, and colitis
- Protects the health of the kidneys
- Reduces the risk of and increases relief from urinary-tract conditions such as bacterial cystitis, interstitial cystitis, and uric-acid kidney stones
- Reduces the risk of gout

- Reduces the risk of and helps in the treatment of rheumatoid arthritis and other autoimmune diseases
- Lowers the risk of osteoporosis and promotes bone growth
- Aids in the prevention and treatment of diabetes
- Reduces hypertension
- May reduce the risk of cancer

Checklist: Are You Overly Acidic?

Put a check mark beside those statements that are true for you.

Lifestyle Factors

o   I do not feel my best when I eat fast foods, fried foods, colas, and desserts.

o   I do not feel my best when I eat red meat or red meat dishes.

o   I do not tolerate acidic condiments like vinegar and lemon juice.

o   I regularly consume processed and refined foods that contain chemical additives.

o   I regularly consume breads and baked goods made with white flour and sugar.

o   I eat few fruits and vegetables.

o   I drink more than one cup of coffee or tea each day.

o   I frequently take ascorbic acid (vitamin C), aspirin, or antibiotics.

o   I do not tolerate alcohol.

o   I have a history of cigarette smoking.

o   I frequently travel by plane.

Performance Indicators

o   I often feel exhausted after vigorous exercise or very physical work.

o   I often experience fatigue and lack of stamina.

o   I run out of breath running up stairs or walking briskly.

o   I am physically and mentally tired after an hour of desk work.

o   I have a tendency to be pessimistic, with little energy to begin new projects.

Physical Indicators

o   I have thin, porous bones.

o   I have poorly developed muscles.

o   I often experience muscle stiffness and soreness.

o   I am over fifty years of age.

Medical History

o   I catch colds or flus frequently.

o   I am susceptible to heartburn, canker sores, food or environmental allergies, and sore throat.

o   I have a history of osteoporosis, arthritis, gout, lung disease, or kidney disease.

Checklist: Are You a High Alkaline Producer?

Performance Indicators

o   I am able to sprint up stairs.

o   I have great physical endurance.

o   I am always on the go and full of energy.

o   I need only a few hours of sleep each night.

o   I am in a position of leadership at work or in the community.

o   I prefer highly active sports and gravitate toward high-stress activities.

o   feel bright and energized after a steak dinner.

o   I am able to digest a wide variety of foods.

o   I feel de-energized after a vegetarian meal.

o   I feel relaxed and healthy while leading a full life.

o   I typically have lots of energy in the midst of intense emotions and high drama.

o   I am able to do desk work for long hours at a time without becoming tired or losing mental clarity.

o   I have an optimistic nature and am always ready to begin something new.

o   I easily maintain an active social life.

o   I rarely get a cold or the flu.

o   I am free of allergies.

Physical Indicators

o   I have a stocky build and a large frame.

o   I am strong and large-boned.

o   I have well-developed muscles.

Now that you have a preliminary understanding of the importance of acid-alkaline balance to peak performance and optimal health, as well as some idea from the checklists of your own functioning in this area, you are ready to decide what to read next.

To learn more about the chemistry of acid and alkaline and how the body regulates this function, read the following section. If you would like to skip this section, you can go to the next chapter to learn how diet, lifestyle, and aging affect acid-alkaline balance.

1

The Chemistry of Acid and Alkaline

All substances in nature can be classified according to their relative acidity or alkalinity. The origin of the word acid is the Latin word "acidus," which means sour or tart. These qualities characterize many of the common acidic substances that we come in contact with, such as the vinegar used in salad dressings, which contain acetic acid; soft drinks, which contain phosphoric acid and carbon dioxide; and black tea, which contains tannic acid. Citric acid is found in grapefruits, oranges, lemons, and limes; and tartaric acid comes from grapes. In contrast, alkaline substances have a bitter taste and feel slippery or smooth on the tongue. A good example is sodium bicarbonate, also known as baking soda, which is used as an antacid.

Several theories were proposed in the late 1800s and early 1900s to explain the chemistry of acid and alkaline substances. While a detailed discussion of these concepts is beyond the scope of this book, it is worth mentioning that the earliest of these theories was developed in 1884, by the Swedish scientist Savant Arrhenius. He limited his theory to water-based solutions and explained that when a substance releases positively charged hydrogen ions (H+) into a solution, an acid is formed. The more hydrogen ions a solution contains, the more acidic it is.

The hydrogen atom (the smallest atom found on Earth) is composed of a nucleus that contains a single positively charged particle called a proton. Outside of the nucleus, the hydrogen atom contains a single negatively charged particle called an electron. (Larger atoms contain more protons and electrons.) The hydrogen ion (H+) consists of only the positively charged nucleus. In contrast, when hydroxide ions (OH–), which are negatively charged molecules of oxygen and hydrogen bonded together, are released into water, they form an alkaline solution. Thus, an alkaline solution contains an excess of electrons.

A second theory of acidity and alkalinity, developed in 1923 by the Danish chemist J. N. Bronsted and the English chemist T. M. Lowry, expanded the concept to include not only water-based solutions but also solids and gases. In doing so, they broadened the definition of acid and alkaline substances beyond hydrogen and hydroxide ions to include many other substances. In their theory, an acid was defined more generally as a proton donor, and an alkaline substance as a proton acceptor.

How Acidity and Alkalinity Are Measured

We have all heard the term pH. It literally refers to the "potential of hydrogen," which is the concentration of hydrogen ions in a given solution. The potential of hydrogen is measured on a scale from 0.00 to 14.00. A ranking above 7.00 indicates that a substance is alkaline, and below 7.00, that it is acid. Pure water has a pH close to neutral, or 7.00. The pH measurement is an extremely sensitive calibration, with an increase or decrease from one whole number to another indicating a tenfold increase or decrease in hydrogen ion concentration. Thus, seemingly small shifts in the pH value of a substance can reflect significant changes in its relative acidity or alkalinity.

How Acidity and Alkalinity Are Neutralized

When acidic and alkaline substances are combined, they neutralize each other. This means that the resulting compound will have a pH closer to the neutral pH of 7.0 than either of the original two substances. A simple example of this occurs when positively charged hydrogen ions (H+) combine with negatively charged hydroxide ions (OH–) to form water (H_2O), a neutral, stable compound. You can also find the end products of acid-alkaline reactions in baked goods, which rise during baking when alkaline ingredients like baking soda are combined with acidic ingredients like lemon juice or sweeteners.

How Acidity and Alkalinity Function Within the Human Body

Our bodies contain trillions of cells, fluid-filled structures that contain many alkaline substances: minerals such as calcium, magnesium, potassium, and sodium, as well as oxygen and bicarbonate. The combination of all of these substances within the cell produces a slightly alkaline intracellular pH of just above 7.00. The cells are also surrounded by fluids that contain alkaline minerals.

All of the metabolic and enzymatic reactions of the body function most efficiently in an alkaline environment. These include energy production, immunity, digestion, and the repair of the body, all of which are necessary for our survival. For example, to produce energy from the nutrients that we ingest in food, a healthy cell requires abundant oxygen, a highly alkaline element. In the presence of oxygen, a series of chemical reactions occurs within the mitochondria or energy-producing factories of the cell: Glucose and other nutrient substances are broken down and converted to adenosine triphosphate (ATP), the universal energy currency of the body. For the body to be able to extract the maximum amount of energy from the food we eat, an abundance of oxygen must be present. Energy production proceeds best, therefore, in a richly alkaline environment.

Not only are the cells of the body alkaline, but the blood that circulates throughout the body must maintain a very narrow range of slightly alkaline pH, 7.35 to 7.45. The constancy of the blood pH is fundamental to the body's ability to maintain a relatively unchanging internal environment. The blood is constantly exposed to a variety of mostly acidic substances (alkaline substances, such as baking soda and a few of the foods we eat, are much less frequently encountered by the body). Various things, from the foods we eat to the stresses in our lives, from the sports we participate in to the pollutants we are exposed to—as well as our own metabolic processes—produce chemicals within the body that are often more acidic than our own slightly alkaline pH. All of these substances are carried within the blood, which transports them to the cells for use as nutrients or carries them away from the cells as waste products.

All of these substances potentially disrupt the healthy pH of the blood. As a result, the body has to have a mechanism to both neutralize and eliminate these substances in order to keep the pH of the blood constant. This is the pH-regulating system. Its importance is illustrated by the fact that a person cannot live more than a few hours if the blood's pH goes below 7.00 or above 8.00. For example, blood with a pH of 6.95, which is only slightly acidic, can lead to coma and even death.

A few compartments of the body, primarily those of the digestive tract, have a pH range that differs from that of the blood. For example, the pH of saliva is 6.0 to 7.5, which is needed to begin the digestion of starches in the mouth. Proteins are much harder to break down than carbohydrates and require an acid environment for their digestion—found in the stomach, which secretes hydrochloric acid. This brings the pH of the stomach down to a highly acidic 1.0 to 3.5.

Once the food leaves the stomach, it must be brought up to an alkaline pH so that the enzymes necessary for further digestion can be activated within the small intestine. The breakdown of nutrients into small particles as well as their absorption occurs in the small intestine. These processes also require an alkaline environment to proceed efficiently. Digestive juices containing sodium and potassium bicarbonate that are secreted by the pancreas into the small intestine have an alkaline pH varying from 8.0 to 9.0. Bile produced by the liver and secreted into the upper part of the small intestine also helps in the process of digestion by breaking down fats. Bile has a pH of 7.8, which is also slightly alkaline. Finally, the intestinal glands, which are located over virtually the entire surface of the small intestine, produce intestinal secretions that have a pH of 7.5 to 8.0.

How the Body Regulates Acid-Alkaline Balance

The pH-regulating system of the body is very complex and is made up of many parts. Within the body, the various parts of our pH-regulating system are carefully orchestrated to work well together. The system includes the alkaline minerals contained both inside and outside the cells, as well as the mineral reserves stored within our bones. We also have three buffer systems in the blood that help to keep its pH constant. In addition, the lungs help to regulate pH by breathing in alkaline oxygen and eliminating acidic waste products in the form of carbon dioxide. Finally, the kidneys eliminate excessive amounts of either acid or alkaline substances from the body through the urine.

The pH-regulating system tends to be healthy and to work efficiently in children and young adults. There are, however, children who have weak buffer systems and tend to become overly acidic early in life as well as some youngsters who are high-alkaline producers and maintain this tendency throughout life. The healthy buffering capability of most young people is due to the robust mineral reserves stored in their bones, healthy buffer systems, and strong lung and kidney function.

However, as people age and experience the mostly acidifying stresses of modern life, the pH-regulating system begins to decline in its efficiency. This decline is a part of the normal aging process and can be accelerated by such factors as strenuous athletic activity or years of acidifying stress or of eating the standard Western diet. As a result, with age, more and more individuals who formerly had good pH balance tend to become overly acidic.

Let's now look briefly at each component of the pH regulating system.

The Mineral Balance Inside and Outside the Cells Helps to Maintain Their Alkaline pH

The minerals that are contained both within the cells and the fluids that surround the cells help to regulate the pH of this microenvironment. These minerals also help to maintain the fluid balance both inside and outside the cells. Minerals, such as sodium, potassium, magnesium, and calcium, are taken into our bodies through the foods we eat and the beverages we drink. Within the body, these minerals take the form of electrolytes, which are mineral salts that dissolve in water and carry an electrical charge. As these minerals move in and out of the cells, they draw fluids with them. Optimal electrolyte and fluid balance allows the cell to absorb nutrients and discharge waste products, as well as maintain its energy level.

Healthy cell membrane function plays an important role in controlling this flow of electrolytes. When the cell membrane is intact, it protects the alkaline pH within the cell. Good digestion also contributes to this process because the breakdown and absorption of food supplies all the cells and their surrounding fluids with the electrolyte minerals and other nutrients required for the buffering process.

The Mineral Reserves Within the Bones Help to Maintain the Alkaline pH of the Blood

Bones are composed of at least eighteen nutrients, many of which are minerals. These include magnesium, manganese, sodium, potassium, zinc, boron, copper, strontium, and calcium, the most publicized of the bone minerals. The bones contain as much as 85 percent of all the phosphorus, 60 percent of the magnesium reserves, and 99 percent of the calcium contained within the body. Most people assume that bone has a solid mineral structure throughout. In actuality, bone is made up of two distinctly different materials: (1) a flexible protein matrix (2) into which are deposited a variety of minerals such as calcium and phosphorus. These minerals provide the bone with tensile strength and rigidity. Thus, its unique structure allows bone to be both flexible and rigid.

Many of the minerals found within the bone are alkaline. While they give bones their strength, they also serve as a reservoir of highly important alkaline minerals, which are capable of buffering acids. Bones are constantly releasing their alkaline minerals to neutralize the acids that we are constantly producing within the body or ingesting in food. Special cells in the bone, called osteoclasts, break down bones, allowing their minerals to be released into the blood as needed for buffering.

The greater the acidity of the body and the weaker the other buffer systems are, the more the bones will be called upon to donate their minerals to keep the body's pH slightly alkaline. When depletion of the bone's mineral reserves occurs over many decades, the result can be osteoporosis, a common disease of the elderly. People who have a tendency toward overacidity may so weaken the structure of their bones, through the loss of alkaline minerals such as calcium that they begin to experience bone fractures by their sixties and seventies.

Three Buffer Systems Maintain the Slightly Alkaline pH of the Blood

The body also regulates pH through its acid-alkaline buffer systems. An acid-alkaline buffer is a solution that contains two or more chemical compounds with the unique ability to prevent radical changes in pH. A buffer limits how much the concentration of hydrogen ions in a solution can increase or decrease when an acid or an alkaline substance is added. For example, if a few drops of lemon juice are added to a glass of water, the pH of the water drops.

However, if the water contains an alkaline compound like sodium bicarbonate, the citric acid in the lemon juice will instantly combine with it, thereby minimizing or preventing any lowering of the pH caused by the addition of the acidic lemon juice. Common buffering compounds used to treat health problems or in the preparation of food include calcium carbonate, sodium bicarbonate, and potassium citrate.

Not surprisingly, the blood contains three different buffer systems. Their complementary action enables the blood to maintain its tightly regulated, slightly alkaline pH of 7.35 to 7.45. These systems are the bicarbonate buffer system, the phosphate buffer system, and the protein buffer system. For example, a highly acidic meal, such as a cheeseburger, French fries, and a cola drink, can cause a surge of acid in the blood, which the body must neutralize. The buffer systems within the blood work very quickly, within one second, to reestablish the blood's normal pH.

The bicarbonate buffer system. Bicarbonate is the body's most important buffering substance and is present in large quantities. The bicarbonate buffer system consists of an acid and an alkaline compound, both of which can be used as buffering agents. The alkaline compound is sodium bicarbonate, while the acid compound is carbonic acid. Working together, they help to neutralize strong acid or alkaline substances that are released into the bloodstream, thereby preventing either a marked rise or fall in the pH of the blood. This system comes into play rapidly as the body is challenged by either acid or alkaline substances, providing a response that can occur within a fraction of a second.

Bicarbonate is also found within the cells of the body and helps to keep both the cells and the extracellular fluids slightly alkaline. Finally, particularly high concentrations of bicarbonate are also produced by the pancreas and secreted as part of the pancreatic digestive juices, whose concentration of bicarbonate is five times greater than that of the blood. As a result, the pancreatic digestive juices have a pH of 8.0. The secretion of these juices is stimulated by the presence of chyme (the mixture of partially digested food and stomach acids) in the small intestine. The pancreas secretes water and bicarbonate, which neutralizes the chyme. When this bicarbonate comes in contact with the hydrochloric acid in the chyme, the resulting reaction produces sodium chloride (table salt) and carbonic acid, which is much weaker than hydrochloric acid. Carbonic acid immediately breaks down into carbon dioxide and water. Carbon dioxide is eventually eliminated from the body by the lungs during exhalation.

This neutralization of the acidic gastric juice produced by the stomach is very important because otherwise the strong acids coming in contact with the surface tissues of the intestine would erode these tissues and could eventually cause ulcers. The bicarbonate excreted by the pancreas also plays another role in digestion, helping to provide the slightly alkaline pH at which pancreatic digestive enzymes are activated.

The phosphate buffer system. The phosphate buffer system acts in a similar manner to the bicarbonate buffer system, containing both acid and alkaline compounds that help to keep the pH of the blood close to neutral. This system also plays a role in helping the kidneys to regulate pH through the excretion of acidic hydrogen ions (H+). The kidneys play an important role in maintaining the pH of the body by eliminating excessive amounts of acidic or alkaline substances through the urine. In addition, the phosphate buffer system also helps to regulate the pH of intracellular fluids, where it is found in high concentrations.

The protein buffer system. The proteins found within the bloodstream and cells are among the most abundant buffering agents found within the body. It is estimated that about 75 percent of all the chemical buffering power of the body fluids resides within the cells because the intracellular proteins act as weak acid buffers. The proteins contained within the cells also provide an important source of buffering for the extracellular fluids. This system acts more slowly since substances must move through the cell membrane in order to be buffered by the proteins contained within the cells. Thus, this system does not provide an immediate response to changes in pH but comes into play after several hours.

Within the bloodstream, hemoglobin, the protein portion of the red blood cell, transports oxygen, an alkaline element, to the tissues. Besides its responsibility as a transport protein, hemoglobin also has a buffering function since it controls the amount of oxygen released into the tissues. For example, during heavy exercise hemoglobin releases larger amounts of oxygen to the tissues. This helps to raise the pH of the tissues since heavy exertion produces acidic waste products that must be buffered; otherwise, these waste products would lower the pH to unhealthy levels.

The Organs of Elimination Help to Return pH to the Normal Range

The lungs and kidneys also play an important role in the regulation of pH. When acid levels rise too high, both of these organs help both to eliminate acid substances from the body and preserve alkaline substances within the body. The reverse occurs if the body becomes too alkaline.

The lungs: Respiratory regulation of acid-alkaline balance. As our organs of respiration, the lungs play a major role in maintaining the normal pH of the blood and tissues. When we breathe in, we inhale the surrounding air, which contains approximately 20 percent oxygen. Oxygen is an alkaline gas that is vital for life since it is used in all the energy-producing chemical reactions of the cells. When we exhale, we breathe out carbon dioxide, an acidic compound that is a waste product produced by all the cells of the body. The lungs help to regulate pH by bringing air and blood into contact so that the acidic carbon dioxide circulating in the blood can be expelled and the alkaline oxygen absorbed by the body. The structure of the lungs allows for maximum exchange of these gases. This exchange of oxygen for carbon dioxide occurs deep within the lungs where the alveoli, or microscopic air sacs, come into contact with tiny blood vessels called capillaries from the pulmonary arteries. Here, the blood and air are separated by only the thinnest of tissues.

When there is a change in pH, the respiratory system is capable of providing a fairly rapid response. While the buffer systems of the blood act within one second, the lungs help to correct pH imbalances within one to two minutes. When the body becomes too acidic, positively charged hydrogen ions have a direct effect on the respiratory center of the brain. This in turn causes ventilation within the lungs to increase four- to fivefold, allowing for more rapid discharge of acidic carbon dioxide, which helps to maintain the slightly alkaline pH of the blood.

Conversely, when the body becomes too alkaline, ventilation decreases, and more carbon dioxide is retained within the body. This causes the pH to drop slightly and, thereby, remain in the normal range. While the lungs cannot completely correct the pH imbalances that occur within the body, they are 50 to 70 percent effective in achieving this goal.

The kidneys: A slow and powerful acid-alkaline regulator. The kidneys' response to changes in pH is the most powerful of all the regulatory systems. Their unique structure allows them to perform the final step in the buffering of excess acidity or alkalinity within the body. The two kidneys sit at the back of the abdominal cavity near the waist. Each kidney contains over 1 million microscopic structural units called nephrons. Each nephron contains tubules (the site of urine formation) and glomeruli (a network of capillaries that filters the blood circulating through the kidneys).

The many waste products of the cells filter from the glomeruli into the tubules, where the regulation of pH takes place. It is via this filtrate that hydrogen ions and organic acids can be excreted from the body through the urine in order to reduce overacidity. The kidneys also retain bicarbonate to help raise the pH. Conversely, it is also the kidneys' job to excrete excessive amounts of alkaline substances when the pH rises too high. The end result is that the kidneys respond to changes of pH within the body by excreting either an acid or alkaline urine. In the process of responding to pH imbalances, urine may have a pH as low as 4.5 or as high as 8.0.

While the kidneys provide a slow correction to pH disturbances, they continue to act until the pH of the body is restored nearly to normal. As a result, the kidneys' correction of acid-alkaline imbalances is total rather than partial and takes from several hours to as long as six days to restore balance. While the kidneys can normally handle a significant amount of acid or alkaline waste products, the production or ingestion of too much acid or alkaline substance can overburden their ability to regulate pH. Serious pH imbalances can then occur.

Summary

All substances can be classified as either acid or alkaline. The human body is slightly alkaline, and has a complex system that works to maintain that balance. All parts of the system, including the mineral balance inside and outside the cells, the mineral reserves within the bones, and three buffer systems in the blood, work together, along with the lungs and the kidneys, to prevent the body from becoming overly acidic. However, some outside factors can alter this favorable balance.

2

How Diet, Lifestyle and Aging Affect Acid-Alkaline Balance

Substances that are too acidic or too alkaline are constantly being produced within the body as a result of the many thousands of chemical reactions that occur on a continual basis. If our buffer systems are working efficiently, these substances are neutralized by our pH-regulating system almost as quickly as they are formed. Unfortunately, most of us begin to experience a decline in the efficient functioning of our pH-regulating system by the time we reach our forties or fifties.

This process is accelerated in many individuals by overexposure to a wide variety of environmental stresses, which tend to expose our bodies to substances that either are highly acidic or create an excessive acid load within the body. With proper education and information, however, we can learn to avoid many of these environmental stresses.

For example, most of the foods in the standard American diet are either highly acidic or acid-forming. In addition, emotional stress, strenuous exercise, long airplane flights, medications, infectious diseases, and certain illnesses as well as the production of our normal metabolic waste products all contribute to acid buildup within the body. This excessive acid load will, over time, deplete the alkaline reserves of most individuals at a much younger age than what we would expect given a normal aging process. For example, constant overacidity depletes the stores of alkaline minerals contained within the bones as well as the ability of the pancreas to produce sufficient bicarbonate-rich digestive juices.

These stresses can lead to a wide range of symptoms due to chronic overacidity. One sign of acidity is feeling noticeably stiff upon arising. Another is feeling either extremely tired or energized after a day of physical exercise. You may find that having red wine with dinner gives you a runny nose or a headache the next day. At least once a month, you have a sore throat.

Overacidity also dramatically increases the frequency of colds, flulike symptoms, allergies, canker sores, heartburn, alternating constipation and diarrhea, insomnia, inflammatory conditions, parasites, fungal conditions, and bone loss. You may also find yourself recovering more slowly from illnesses, cuts, minor surgery, or even normal physical exertion.

The Highly Acidic Standard American Diet

The typical American diet is composed mainly of foods that are either highly acidic in their chemical makeup or, once eaten, cause an acidic reaction within the body. These foods include red meat, poultry, dairy products, most fruits, nuts, refined sugar, corn sweeteners, chocolate, refined flour products, soft drinks, beer, wine, coffee, and black tea. There are many reasons why these foods tend to be acidic. Many of them contain large amounts of acidic minerals such as sulfur, phosphorus, chlorine, and iodine. Some of these foods also contain acids such as the carbon dioxide used to create the carbonation in soft drinks and beer, the tannic acid found in black tea, and the acetic acid found in vinegar. Examples of acids found in fruits are the malic acid in apples and citric acid contained in oranges, lemons, limes, and grapefruits.

Some of these foods also cause an acidic reaction within the body. For example, red meat, dairy products, and wheat all contain tough and difficult-to-digest proteins such as the casein found in milk and the gluten found in wheat. When these foods are ingested, the stomach must secrete large amounts of hydrochloric acid in order to begin the breakdown of these proteins. This puts a significant stress on the pancreas, liver, and small intestine, which must then produce copious amounts of highly alkaline digestive juices and bile to neutralize the excess acid produced by the stomach. Other foods, such as coffee and alcohol, also trigger excessive acid production by the stomach.

In addition, as food is metabolized within the body, it is converted into a number of acidic waste products such as uric acid, lactic acid, and acetic acid. These acids will lower the pH of body fluids and must be neutralized by the buffer systems contained within the blood; their residues must then be eliminated from the body. Furthermore, acidic by-products derived from the sulfur, chlorine, and phosphorus in foods produce toxic acids such as sulfuric, phosphoric, and hydrochloric acid, which must also be neutralized to avoid damaging the kidneys and other organs of the body. When the liver's ability to detoxify is impaired, many toxic and highly acidic by-products are formed. These acidic by-products must also be neutralized and eliminated from the body.

Finally, many people are allergic to the proteins found in a variety of foods, including dairy products, wheat, peanuts, corn, soybeans, and the milk and nuts used in the preparation of certain chocolate products. Food allergies cause an acidic, inflammatory reaction in sensitive individuals. Some individuals are also sensitive or intolerant to various foods. Common examples are the sugars found in milk (lactose) or fruit (fructose) and the amines found in tomatoes, oranges, wine, chocolate, and Parmesan cheese. Individuals with these sensitivities either find these foods irritating to their systems or lack the enzymes to digest them, thereby leading to overacidity. Many of these same foods also tend to aggravate autoimmune conditions such as rheumatoid arthritis. The inflammation that results from these conditions causes the production of acidic chemicals within the body that must be constantly buffered if the blood is to remain at a slightly alkaline pH.

In summary, overacidity caused by the normal ingestion and breakdown of foods as well as toxic by-products caused by foods can greatly stress our buffering capability. Whether these foods are highly acidic or cause an acid reaction within the body, they must all be neutralized and any acid residues from the food eliminated from the body to keep the pH of the blood slightly alkaline.

Unfortunately, most people eat almost exclusively these highly acidic or acid-forming foods and skimp on foods that are less acidic and more alkaline such as vegetables, starches, whole-grain products (non-gluten-containing), beans and peas, seafood, eggs, and a few fruits like melons and papayas (a chart listing the exact pH of various foods can be found in part 2 of this book in the chapter on the alkaline power diet). These foods are strikingly similar to those found in the Mediterranean diet, which medical authorities currently consider one of the most healthful diets on the planet. The Mediterranean diet has been linked to a lower incidence of such life-threatening illnesses as heart disease and cancer. It is worth noting that this diet is much less acidic than the standard American one.

The prevalence of highly acidic foods in the typical American diet is so overwhelming that our children begin to experience wear and tear on their buffering capability practically at birth. It is common to see very young children sucking on a bottle filled with highly acidic fruit juice. Three- and four-year-olds can commonly be seen drinking highly acidic cola drinks and eating hamburgers. If you look inside the lunch box of any American child or teenager, you are likely to see many different types of highly acidic processed foods like pizza, candy bars, cookies, potato chips, and sandwiches made from white bread and processed meats.

What is lacking in our children's meals are enough of the highly nutritious, less acidic, more alkaline foods like fresh vegetables, legumes, starches, and fish. This dietary pattern has been confirmed in a number of research studies. One such study, published in the Journal of the American Dietetic Association, examined the diet during a twenty-four-hour period of nearly 1800 second- and fifth-graders in New York State. On the day they were surveyed, it was found that 40 percent did not eat vegetables except for potatoes or tomato sauce, and 36 percent ate at least four different types of snack foods. The study also found that 16 percent of the fifth-graders did not eat breakfast. Another study, reported in the same journal, found that children who did not eat breakfast had a lower intake of many essential vitamins and minerals, including alkaline minerals like calcium and magnesium. In other words, the children who skipped breakfast did not make up their nutritional deficiencies at other meals.

Adults in our society do not fare much better, given the enormous quantities of highly acidic coffee, beer, wine, fruit juice, fast foods, processed food, frozen entrées, and convenience foods that many of us eat. Many people consume highly acidic coffee and cola drinks for their caffeine content, to energize them and keep them awake. Most of us eat fast foods and convenience foods to help us manage our busy lives, and drink alcoholic beverages at night to help us relax. It is, therefore, no surprise that by midlife most of us have begun to wear out our buffering capability and are beginning to suffer the ill effects of overacidity on our performance and health. Only the peak performers who are high-alkaline producers can survive and even thrive on the standard American diet.

The statistics supplied by the Economic Research Service of the USDA confirm this imbalance in the American diet. I added up the number of pounds of highly acidic or acid-forming foods that the average American eats per year, and compared this with the average yearly intake of less acid, more alkaline foods. The ratio was an astonishing 17:3 in favor of acidic or acid-forming foods. This predominance of acid-forming foods in the American diet puts an enormous stress on the buffering capability of many Americans to neutralize all of this acid.

One reason for this imbalance in our diet is that highly acidic foods are far more available and much more highly promoted through advertising than more alkaline foods. The majority of space in the supermarket is devoted to highly acidic foods because these foods tend to have long shelf lives while many of the more alkaline foods are highly perishable.

The mainstays of fast food—hamburgers, pizza, fried chicken, prepackaged wedges of apple pie, and colas—are primarily composed of highly acidic ingredients. American corporations involved in producing packaged foods that have long shelf lives or in selling fast foods are among the largest advertisers in the United States. Thus, while we are deluged with ads for highly acidic food products, we rarely see a promotional campaign for more alkaline foods like melons or papayas.

The following subsections describe the main categories of common foods and their general acid content.

Protein

The Western diet is relatively high in protein, ranging from 50 to 100 grams (g) per day (about 2 to 3½ oz.). Of this amount, the body can comfortably process only 40 to 60 g. You can see how easy it is to reach this amount when you look at the protein content of various foods. For example, an 8 oz. sirloin steak or serving of lamb or pork contains between 35 and 40 g of protein. A similar sized serving of chicken or turkey contains between 15 and 20 g of protein, while 8 oz. of fish contains an amazing 40 to 50 g. In addition, dairy products, eggs, and even vegetarian sources of protein such as beans, peas, seeds, nuts, and whole grains can greatly add to our daily protein intake.

While the body needs an adequate intake of protein each day to build and repair tissue, any excess must be broken down and then excreted. By-products of this process are sulfuric acid and phosphoric acid. Protein is eventually converted to uric acid, which is eliminated in the urine.

The amount of protein a person consumes can significantly affect acid-alkaline balance. This was demonstrated in a study, published in the American Journal of Clinical Nutrition. Volunteers were fed various protein-based diets consisting of either 49, 95, or 120 g of protein per day. The researchers measured hydrogen ion excretion in the urine to study the effect of protein intake on acidity. While the low-protein diet caused only a small increase in hydrogen ions in the urine, the hydrogen ion content increased thirtyfold with the high-protein diet. This increase reflected the body's need to eliminate the excessive amount of acid generated by the protein consumed to enable the pH of the blood to remain slightly alkaline.

A high intake of protein can further stress our acid-alkaline balance by accelerating the loss of alkaline minerals such as calcium from the body. There are many studies in the medical literature documenting this effect. For example, in a study published in the Journal of Nutrition, women were given a diet of either 46 or 123 g of protein a day for sixty days. The higher protein diet resulted in a doubling of calcium lost in the urine.

Refined Flour and Sugar

Another major source of dietary acid is refined flour products like white bread, pasta, crackers, cookies, donuts, and other pastries that are eaten by the great majority of us throughout the day. Many of these foods are also highly sugared, which further adds to their acid content. White flour is a simple carbohydrate. During the refining process, a significant portion of the vitamins, minerals, and fiber are lost; what remains is predominantly starch.

When sugar is processed, all vitamins and minerals are removed; what remains is the simple sugar molecule, glucose. Refined flour and sugar enter the system rapidly and break down quickly, producing acids. Lactic acid is one highly acidic end product of glucose metabolism, occurring particularly during periods when oxygen levels are reduced within the body. Lactic acid must be buffered to keep the pH of the blood slightly alkaline. Furthermore, these foods do not provide the alkaline minerals necessary to buffer the acids that they generate.

Fats

For most Americans, fat composes 30 to 40 percent of their dietary intake. While the pH of fats cannot be measured because they do not go into an aqueous solution, fats are metabolized into acidic breakdown products. In addition, certain fats, such as those found in red meat and dairy products, contain arachidonic acid. Arachidonic acid is converted within the body to a variety of inflammatory substances such as leukotrienes and prostaglandins, which are powerful triggers of inflammation within various tissues.

For example, leukotrienes can trigger asthmatic episodes, while prostaglandin production can worsen inflammatory-like rheumatoid arthritis and endometriosis. These inflammatory reactions cause acidic reactions within the affected tissues. Those suffering from diabetes are particularly prone to acidosis since they experience the breakdown of fats into substances called ketones that have an acidifying effect on the body.

Beverages

Many popular beverages including coffee, colas, wine, beer, and virtually all fruit juices are quite acidic. Coffee has a pH that varies from 4.9 to 5.2, beer has a pH ranging between 4.0 and 5.0, diet soft drinks are around 3.0, and colas, 2.6. Since Americans drink more soft drinks than water, these drinks contribute significantly to the high level of acidity in the American diet. The acidity is partly due to the carbon dioxide content of these beverages, which gives them their bubbles. Soft drinks also contain such acidic ingredients as sugar and flavoring and coloring agents. Fruit juices tend to be as acidic as soft drinks. For example, apple juice has a pH of 3.4, grapefruit juice has a pH of 2.9 to 3.4, and lime and lemon juice are very acidic, with a pH range of 1.8 to 2.6.

On the positive side, some fruit juices like orange juice and apple juice are excellent sources of alkaline minerals like potassium. However, these fruit juices may be poorly tolerated by overly acidic individuals, who are sensitive to the low pH of these drinks. Such people may be able to enjoy these fruit juices when they are consumed in combination with foods having a higher pH that are also rich sources of alkaline minerals, such as many vegetables, grains, beans, and peas.

Flavoring Agents and Additives

Vinegar, a common flavoring agent in salad dressings, mustards, mayonnaise, and marinades, contains acetic acid. The acid content of commercial vinegars is clearly marked on the bottle at 5 percent, and these products have a pH ranging from 2.4 to 3.5. Acetic acid gives vinegar its tart and sour taste. The majority of processed and packaged foods usually contain added salt and sugar, which are both acidifying substances. If marketed as sugar-free, processed foods probably contain artificial sweeteners such as aspartame or saccharin, which are also acidic.

Lifestyle and Acid-Alkaline Balance

Many of the standard components of modern life act to increase the acid level of the body. These include stress, exercise, airplane travel, and the use of medications.

The Acidifying Effect of Stress

When we are under physical and mental stress, we use more nutrients and generate more acidic waste products than the body can process and dispose of rapidly. Strong emotions of any kind increase acidity: Anger, fear, hostility, and even excitement generate acids within the body because they reduce oxygenation and blood flow to the tissues and increase muscle tension.

People who are experiencing stress and are overly acidic may also be more prone to infections. Research conducted at Carnegie-Mellon University studied the relationship between emotions and depressed immunity. The researchers found that people who were currently involved in stressful personal relationships or experiencing problems with their job had a higher risk of developing the common cold, a condition related to overacidity.

Exercise

As a person exercises, oxygen is consumed, and lactic acid and carbon dioxide, among other waste products, are created. Studies have shown that the more vigorous the exercise, the more these acids accumulate, which results in a decrease in the pH of the muscles. This hampers energy production within muscle tissue and can significantly limit athletic endurance and performance. In extreme cases of acid buildup, the muscle, finally, can no longer function. We have all seen an athlete unable to continue sprinting or lifting a weight due to muscle failure caused by the buildup of excess acids.

Frequent Airplane Travel

Most people are unaware that spending hours in an airplane increases acidity within the body. This is because the stale, recirculated air in the passenger compartment of a commercial plane has a lower concentration of oxygen. At the same time, the confinement of several hundred people in a small area causes the level of carbon dioxide in the air to increase. In addition, international flights still permit cigarette smoking, which further depletes the oxygen content of the plane's cabin as well as adding many acidic chemicals to the recirculating air.

Medications

Many over-the-counter medications are acidifying, including aspirin (acetylsalicylic acid) and the sweet-tasting cough syrups that millions of Americans use to treat colds, flus, and bronchitis. Even an important nutritional supplement like vitamin C (ascorbic acid) is acidic. There have also been documented cases in the medical literature of acidic reactions to antibiotics.

Medical Conditions

Some medical conditions also increase the acid level of the body. Most of these are chronic or traumatic, but it is important to know how they affect acid-alkaline balance, so that steps can be taken to correct imbalances.

Respiratory acidosis. Diseases such as emphysema and chronic bronchitis can lead, over time, to severe lung damage, which can impair one's ability to fully oxygenate the body through respiration. At the same time, the lungs are unable to efficiently eliminate carbon dioxide, which normally occurs during exhalation. This can cause a dangerous condition called respiratory acidosis in which the blood pH begins to drop. If not corrected, this condition can lead to significant impairment and death. Acute respiratory infections, like severe pneumonia, can also lead to respiratory acidosis and must be aggressively treated.

Metabolic acidosis. Many chronic health conditions can eventually lead to a condition called metabolic acidosis in which acidic waste products accumulate in the body. For example, with chronic kidney disease, the ability to eliminate waste products through the urine is impaired. Acute adrenal insufficiency is associated with severe electrolyte and fluid imbalances. Large amounts of hydrogen and potassium are lost in the urine, resulting in metabolic acidosis.

Metabolic acidosis can also occur in severe liver disease since the liver is no longer able to perform its detoxifying function efficiently. This leads to the accumulation of highly acidic and toxic by-products of metabolism. In diabetic ketoacidosis, the cells are not able to utilize glucose in the blood to produce energy. In this state of starvation, fat and protein are broken down to meet the body's energy needs. However, this breakdown can occur faster than the body is able to use these fuels, and their acidic residues build up in the blood, causing its pH to drop. This condition can also occur with severe diarrhea from any cause when alkaline minerals are lost through the digestive tract.

Burns and surgery. Burns and surgery cause physical damage to tissues, resulting in decreased blood flow and oxygenation to the affected areas. In severe cases, metabolic acidosis can develop. Acidosis may be aggravated in burn patients who have suffered from smoke inhalation, resulting in impaired lung function. The ability of surgical patients to regulate pH may be further compromised if they are prescribed diuretics, enemas, or laxatives, all of which accelerate the loss of alkaline minerals from the body.

The Ability to Regulate pH Diminishes with Age

The aging of the lungs, kidneys, and pancreas affects our ability to maintain acid-alkaline balance as we grow older. Children and young adults tend to have excellent functional capability of these vital organs. However, between the ages of thirty-five and sixty, the ability to buffer begins to decline in most people. While this is due, in part, to the normal aging process, the decline in our buffering capability is accelerated by the constant wear and tear caused by the standard American diet, stress, exposure to pollutants, and a variety of other factors.

With advancing age, our lungs' ability to take in oxygen declines significantly. The intake of oxygen with each breath declines by about 1 percent a year on average. Oxygen intake in men peaks at about age twenty-five and in women at age twenty. By age seventy, oxygen intake may be reduced by half. This is due to the loss of elasticity of the lung tissue and, even, reduced mobility of the rib cage, which can make breathing more of an effort.

The result of these changes is that the body receives less alkalinizing oxygen and expels less acidifying carbon dioxide. Chronic exposure to pollutants such as formaldehyde, ammonia, and other toxic chemicals may cause lung irritation and asthma. Cigarette smoking increases the risk of serious lung diseases such as bronchitis and emphysema, which further reduce the pH-regulating function of the lungs and accelerate their aging.

The kidney's ability to regulate pH also declines with age. After the age of forty, the ability of the kidneys to filter waste from the blood diminishes by about 1 percent per year. After midlife, the ability of the pancreas to secrete bicarbonate begins to decline. There is also a drop in production of secretin, the hormone that stimulates the pancreas to release bicarbonate.

High-Alkaline Producers: The Exceptions to the Rule

Approximately 6 to 8 percent of the population tend to be high-alkaline producers. In contrast to the majority, these people often maintain excellent buffering capability well into old age. They usually have excellent lung capacity and digestive function as well as large reserves of alkaline minerals within their bones, which they can draw on for decades longer than the average person. The ability of these individuals to remain slightly alkaline allows them to outperform all of their more acidic peers. In fact, these people actually thrive on the acidic stresses of our modern world.

High-alkaline producers are the only group who can withstand the effects of the highly acidic standard American diet, the environmental pollutants, and the level of physical and emotional stress that most of us are subjected to in our daily lives. They require hard endurance exercise nearly every day to create lactic acid and burn off some energy. They will also gravitate to a personal and professional lifestyle filled with excitement and even danger. These people do not usually start their day by meditating.

Most of the role models of our society, including top athletes, celebrities, business people, and politicians, tend to be high-alkaline producers. Their strong and resilient physiologies allow them to excel and outperform their peers in almost any activity or endeavor. They rarely get ill since the ability to maintain an alkaline pH within the body is necessary for immunity, structural repair, digestive function, and healthy metabolic function in general.

Because they age more slowly, many of these individuals look younger than their age. In their later years, they tend to lead far more active lives than their more acidic contemporaries. Senior citizens who remain highly alkaline are able to lift weights, climb mountains, and run marathons at age eighty with a body that looks decades younger. Photographs of naturally alkaline older men and women sometimes appear in fitness and health magazines. These magazines are read by much younger individuals who see these elders as role models and hope to emulate them when they reach the same age. When these hearty individuals do seek medical help, it is usually not for problems related to overacidity.

Older individuals with alkaline constitutions are able to stay independent and engaged in life. Unlike their more acidic peers, who are unable to live without assistance, either in nursing and retirement homes or from their children, they are more likely to maintain their own homes in their seventies, eighties, and even nineties. Advertisements for cruise ships often feature pictures of these energetic oldsters, dancing aboard ship after having consumed a gigantic buffet dinner of rich foods that people with weaker buffering capabilities could not even conceive of eating.

Many high-alkaline producers often continue to work to an advanced age and continue to pursue all their interests and hobbies, stay up on world events, and enjoy a wide circle of friends. These people defy the law of diminishing expectations. This is not to say that people with alkaline constitutions are immortal, but they are able to retain a tremendous edge in their performance capabilities.

Summary

As we age, our ability to maintain a slightly alkaline balance in our cells and tissues diminishes. All too many factors in modern life, including the standard American diet, also affect acid-alkaline balance in the body. Our diet is high in acidic and acid-creating foods, and the fast pace of life today also increases acidity. Some people are naturally high-alkaline producers, and this characteristic helps them to maintain the peak-performance traits described in the next section.

3

Acid-Alkaline Balance and Peak Performance

The ability to maintain acid-alkaline balance has an amazing effect on five important peak-performance traits: physical vitality and stamina; career performance; mental clarity and acuity; the ability to get along with other people and optimism and vision. This chapter will explain how performing at your best is related to your body's ability to maintain a healthy, slightly alkaline state.

Physical Vitality and Stamina

Some people have jobs that require muscular exertion. To be able to perform their work in a competent manner, they need physical energy, strength, and stamina. I see people performing these jobs on a daily basis: gas and electric repair crews, phone line repair crews, fire fighters and police officers rushing to an emergency, gardeners, farmers, construction workers, and road maintenance crews. Professional dancers and athletes must also be exceptionally physically fit to do their work. None of these people can sustain their careers over a long period of time without being able to maintain their body's slightly alkaline pH.

For example, professional dancers routinely engage in an activity that produces a great deal of acid. Rigorous daily practice and frequent performances constantly produce lactic acid within the muscles. While dancers in their twenties and thirties have the buffering capability to handle this acidic load, the capability to keep the body slightly alkaline in the face of this physical exertion diminishes with age. It is rare to see a dancer perform beyond the age of fifty, when most dancers can no longer keep up with the physical demands of their profession and have sustained too many injuries to continue.

Similarly, professional and other highly trained athletes must have the strong buffering capability necessary to prevent muscle fatigue and maintain the stamina and endurance needed for endless practice sessions and frequent competitive events or regular season games and playoffs. The extraordinary level of performance of great athletes has to be supported, in part, by world class buffer systems.

Most individuals whose jobs require them to do physical work are unable to maintain their physical prowess well into old age. This is because they lose their ability to regulate pH efficiently beginning in midlife or even younger. At this point, physical symptoms of overacidity—such as muscular fatigue, reduced endurance, stiffness, joint pain, and slower recovery from injury or exertion—begin to take their toll, causing many individuals to retire or change their careers to one that is less physically demanding.

The same phenomenon often happens to individuals who have spent years participating in vigorous physical activities such as bodybuilding, jogging, downhill skiing, handball, racquetball, and squash. Most of these sports are pursued by young, vigorous, alkaline individuals. As people begin to reach their forties and fifties, the dropout rate from these sports becomes significant, often for the same reasons that people leave physically demanding jobs.

The accumulation of acids within the muscles and joints begins to cause too much physical discomfort and muscular fatigue for them to continue participating. Most people as they age switch to less physically demanding sports like golf, walking, and relaxed swimming, which are slower paced, more aerobic, and, therefore, less acid producing.

How Overacidity Restricts Physical Energy And Stamina

Let's look at the mechanism of how overacidity restricts physical energy and stamina. Muscle tissue contains several specific buffer systems, including the proteins carnosine and anserine. In resting muscle tissue, these two proteins act as powerful buffering agents. At a neutral pH of 7, they contribute as much as 20 to 30 percent of the buffering action, according to a study published in the *Archives of Biochemistry and Biophysics*. Phosphate contained within the muscle tissue is also an effective buffer. Finally, sodium bicarbonate provides only about 5 to 10 percent of the muscle's buffering capability.

When a person exercises vigorously, glycogen (a form of stored glucose or sugar in the muscles) is burned for energy. By-products of this process are lactic acid and pyruvic acid. As these acids accumulate, the pH of the muscle tissue drops, which begins to hinder muscular activity since these tissues function best, like the rest of the body, with a slightly alkaline pH.

Overacidity causes muscles to become fatigued. One reason this occurs was discussed in a research article published in the British Journal of Sports Medicine. This study found that the accumulation of acids within the muscle limits production of the energy molecule ATP (adenosine triphosphate). It also inhibits the activity of muscle fibers, which impairs the mechanisms by which muscles contract. The body does this to protect the muscles from further physical activity, which would cause the muscles to become even more acidic.

Other studies have confirmed these findings. For example, a study conducted at the Institute of Work Physiology in Oslo, Norway, and published in the Journal of Applied Physiology had volunteers exercise repeatedly for periods of one minute on a treadmill or stationary bicycle. The pH of their blood and muscles became significantly more acidic with this exertion. Another study, conducted at Children's Hospital of San Francisco and published in the Journal of Clinical Investigation, showed that with both intermittent and sustained exercise, the more intense the activity, the faster acid accumulates.

Using Alkalinizing Agents To Enhance Physical Performance

The role that buffering plays in supporting physical energy has primarily been studied in the area of sports performance. Researchers have focused on the use of alkalinizing agents as ergogenic aids, substances that increase the potential for accomplishing a given task and improving performance. In these studies, volunteers are given an alkaline substance such as sodium bicarbonate and then asked to perform an intense physical exercise for a short duration of time, such as sprinting or cycling for two or three minutes. Researchers then measure the degree to which a reduction in acidity will increase the time it takes for muscle exhaustion to occur.

The interest in alkalinizing agents to enhance sports performance goes back many decades. One early study, published in the German Weekly Medical Journal, found that when runners were given an acidifying agent, they became exhausted more quickly than those who were not. In contrast, giving athletes an alkalinizing agent before endurance running or bicycling extended their performance by 30 to 100 percent and reduced their recovery time after physical exhaustion had occurred.

Three different alkalinizing agents have been researched for their beneficial effect on athletic performance: sodium bicarbonate, sodium citrate, and sodium phosphate. While not all of the studies have been positive in their results, most of them suggest that alkalinization is a very powerful tool in enhancing athletic performance.

Sodium bicarbonate. Researchers have learned that sodium bicarbonate buffers muscular acidity indirectly. A study published in the Canadian Journal of Pharmacology found that sodium bicarbonate works by increasing the alkalinity of the blood, rather than entering the muscle cells and directly buffering the acid contained within the muscle tissue. The increased alkalinity of the blood creates a pH gradient between the blood and the more acidic muscle tissue. This gradient causes the acids to be drawn out of the muscle, which then allows them to be neutralized. Another study, published in Clinical Science, reported that muscle biopsies done on athletes also found that pH changes in the blood with alkalinization reflected changes occurring within the muscle.

Subsequent research focused on the potential benefits that sodium bicarbonate loading could produce on extending performance time before muscles reach exhaustion. All of these studies tested athletic performance over a relatively short period of time. While some of these studies have shown that alkalinizing with sodium bicarbonate significantly improved performance, others found this effect to be limited.

Studies published in the British Journal of Sports Medicine and Medicine and Science in Sports and Exercise found bicarbonate loading to be beneficial. The first study used twenty-three volunteers to participate in six trials on a cycle ergometer. Each trial consisted of ten 10-second sprints with a 50-second recovery time allowed between each sprint. A prior pilot study had established that these 10-second sprints would result in fatigue as well as a decline in "peak power." The six trials were double-blind, with the participants ingesting either sodium bicarbonate or a placebo prior to beginning each trial. The trials using sodium bicarbonate produced a higher level of exertional output than those using the placebo.

The second study examined the benefits of sodium bicarbonate loading on the racing times of six male varsity middle-distance runners at a university in Canada. These runners participated in an 800-meter race, an event in which fatigue normally results from the accumulation of lactic acid within the muscles. Sodium bicarbonate loading enabled five of the six participants to improve their running time by an average of 2.9 seconds. This represented a distance of 19 meters, which, the authors noted, in an 800-meter race could be the difference between first and last place.

A further study, published in the International Journal of Sports Medicine, studied the effect that alkalinizing with sodium bicarbonate had on eleven volunteers both before, during, and after five 1-minute sprints on a stationary bicycle. While the volunteers were allowed to take a 1-minute rest between the first four bouts, the final sprint was performed until the subjects became fatigued to the point that they could not maintain their cycling rate. The use of sodium bicarbonate improved the performance time during the final bout by 42 percent in comparison to the same bout done using a placebo.

Finally, in a study published in the journal Ergonomics, seven healthy males ran to exhaustion on a treadmill. Treatment with sodium bicarbonate postponed time to exhaustion by 17 percent, while the acidic compound ammonium chloride shortened the time it took volunteers to become exhausted by 19 percent.

One drawback in applying these findings to everyday exercise and sports routines is that most of the studies used very high doses of sodium bicarbonate to optimize athletic performance. Volunteers were usually given a single dose of sodium bicarbonate at the level of 300 mg/kg of body weight. In a 150-pound man, this would be nearly four teaspoons of sodium bicarbonate. Given that the normal dosage is one-half to one teaspoon, it is no surprise that many of these individuals suffered from intestinal upset and diarrhea.

Sodium citrate. Sodium citrate is a buffering agent that is sometimes used in place of sodium bicarbonate since it has the same buffering capacity but does not cause diarrhea, a common side effect of sodium bicarbonate. Historically, certain fruit juices, which are high in potassium citrate and alkaline salts of citric acid, have been used to raise blood pH. Studies done in the 1930s found that these drinks improved performance in events ranging from 100- to 400-meter swimming sprints to endurance cycling and running.

However, results of more recent studies using sodium citrate have been mixed. One study, published in the European Journal of Applied Physiology, examined the effect of sodium citrate when volunteers cycled for twenty minutes on a stationary bicycle. While there was a measurable increase in blood pH, the sodium citrate did not improve performance during this strenuous exercise.

Sodium phosphate. The mineral phosphorus helps to buffer acids that accumulate within muscle tissue during heavy exercise. Phosphorus produces its beneficial effect in several ways. It is needed for the production of an enzyme called 2,3-diphosphoglycerate (2,3-DPG), which is found in red blood cells. Red blood cells transport oxygen in the blood to the tissues, and 2,3-DPG insures that oxygen, an important alkalinizing agent, is delivered to the muscles. It reduces the affinity that hemoglobin, the carrier molecule in red blood cells, has for oxygen, so oxygen is more available to the tissues. Phosphorus promotes energy production within the cells, functioning together with the B vitamins. It also improves the production and use of glycogen, a sugar that is a ready source of energy in the muscles.

Because the standard American diet contains plentiful amounts of meat and dairy products, which contain large amounts of phosphorus, most people are far from deficient. However, athletes may need especially high amounts of this mineral, since studies have shown that muscles lose phosphorus into the bloodstream during periods of intense physical exertion. The more a person exercises, the more phosphorus is needed by the body. Endurance athletes, such as marathon runners, will have low levels of phosphorus immediately after participating in an athletic event.

One study, published in the British Medical Journal, found that sixteen of the thirty-eight men who collapsed during a six-year period of the Great North Runs had significantly lower phosphate levels than those individuals who successfully completed those races. Another study, published in Muscle and Nerve, found that weight training also causes the loss of phosphorus from muscle tissues. Loss of phosphorus can impair buffering within the muscle tissue and limit the amount of oxygen delivered to the muscle cells.

Phosphorus is given to athletes in a buffered form, sodium phosphate. The sports performance benefits of phosphate loading have been studied, with mixed results. In one study, published in the Journal of Laboratory and Clinical Medicine, six volunteers received infusions of a phosphate-based drug (Didronel) plus fructose-phosphate as well as fructose-phosphate infusions alone. The researchers measured levels of 2,3-DPG and cardiopulmonary (heart-lung) function at three 5-minute intervals as the participants exercised on a stationary bicycle. They found that with either treatment, 2,3-DPG levels increased and the volunteers were able to perform a comparable workload and use the same amount of oxygen without the heart having to work as hard.

However, a later study, conducted at the Human Performance Laboratory at Old Dominion University and published in Medicine and Science in Sports and Exercise, gave volunteers 1000 mg of tribasic sodium phosphate four times daily for six days. This resulted in increased blood levels of phosphate and increased oxygen uptake; however, it did not improve their performance when they competed in a five-mile run.

Alkalinizing Agents and Recreational Sports

While buffering agents have been researched to help serious athletes gain a competitive edge in their field, no one has focused on the benefit that buffering can produce when used in much smaller doses for individuals engaged in everyday sports and athletic activities. I have found alkalinizing agents like sodium and potassium bicarbonate to be tremendously helpful in reducing fatigue, muscle stiffness, and achiness when taken either during or after a long hike, bicycling, playing tennis, or a day on the golf course (carrying your bag, not using a cart).

The use of alkalinizing agents may be particularly beneficial to weekend warriors, especially those in the baby-boomer age group. They often tend to balance their intense work schedules with aggressive, acid-producing exercise. Recovery from such hard exertion can sometimes be slow, due to the production of acid within the muscles. Instead of the ergogenic use of sodium bicarbonate, which entails using a single and very substantial dose for a quick performance boost, most of us would benefit from taking more moderate doses periodically during an athletic event or on a day of strenuous physical activity.

You may find it useful to take moderate amounts of an alkalinizing agent before, during, and after an athletic event to reduce or prevent soreness and to increase endurance and stamina. My alkaline savvy friends take a container full of an alkalinizing agent to sip on periodically during an athletic event or outing. The constant intake of small amounts of alkaline liquid, such as one-half to one teaspoon of sodium bicarbonate (baking soda) or as a dilute solution of sodium and potassium bicarbonate (ranging from a 3:1 to a 4:1 ratio of sodium to potassium, depending on your tolerance for potassium), helps ward off fatigue caused by acid buildup due to the physical exertion. This will help you remain much more energized during an event than eating an acidic energy bar or consuming highly acidic soft drinks, both of which add to the acid load and can subject you to a significant energy letdown.

In addition, anti-inflammatory digestive enzymes should also be taken prior to and/or following strenuous physical exertion to prevent stiffness and soreness from occurring. See my book for digestive health for specific recommendations.

Stressful Careers and the Alkaline Constitution

The necessity of maintaining an alkaline pH is important not just for sports performance but also for many other careers and endeavors that involve arduous schedules, stressful work conditions, long hours, and frequent travel demands. Examples of such careers include emergency room physicians and nurses, upper and middle-managers of corporations, salespeople, investment bankers and brokers, and management consultants, as well as touring entertainers and musicians. These professions do not necessarily demand muscular strength, but they do require a high level of physical energy and stamina. High-alkaline producers have the edge here, just as they do in sports performance. Let's look at a few exceptional examples of individuals in unusually high-profile careers for which being a high alkaline producer is a virtual necessity.

Queen Victoria had the longest reign of any monarch in English history. She exemplified the physical stamina typical of high-alkaline producers. Victoria survived tremendous political upheavals and setbacks, including being the target of seven assassination attempts. She outlived her husband by several decades, and, by the time she died in 1901 and left the throne to her son, Edward VIII, he was already fifty-nine.

In addition to her obvious physical stamina and fortitude in the face of adversity, Queen Victoria also demonstrated her alkaline constitution by giving birth to nine children, a process that puts tremendous stress on the alkaline mineral reserves of the mother. Not only does a fetus grow and develop from the nourishment it derives from its mother's diet, but it also will draw down on the alkaline mineral reserves contained within the mother's bones if her dietary intake is inadequate. This is one reason why women often feel depleted after pregnancy. Only strong alkaline women like Queen Victoria can sustain nine full-term pregnancies without impairing their vitality and exhausting their reserves.

Similarly, great physical stamina is required to hold many of the highest posts in government. The president of the United States has a job that is arduous, stressful, and physically demanding at a level that few people can even comprehend. Presidents have to be high-alkaline producers to maintain the energy, resistance to disease, and ability to recover from injury needed to handle the stresses and physical demands inherent in this job. Another job that requires an alkaline constitution is secretary of state. Individuals holding this position must constantly participate in many acid-producing activities.

In our era of shuttle diplomacy, they are required to travel frequently, often facing a grueling work and social schedule upon arrival at their destination. The secretary of state is required to attend formal state dinners and cocktail parties, which usually serve only rich, acid-producing foods and beverages. Their high-stress work involves daily meetings with various heads of state and other decision makers, each dealing with difficult international issues and tense diplomatic situations. Without superb buffering capability, the people in these positions could not function effectively. Recent presidents of the United States have also exemplified their strong alkaline constitution by living well into their 90's.

Like U.S. presidents, CEOs are the lords of the American corporations. Their job may be almost as stressful and demanding as that of our political president. This is particularly true for entrepreneurs who have grown their companies from scratch. High-alkaline producers make the best entrepreneurs, since this job requires staying power, stamina, and most importantly, physical endurance. With no guaranteed paycheck, entrepreneurs must be able to withstand the risks and frustrations that occur when one is trying to build an enterprise. There is perhaps no better example of such a personality type than Richard Branson, founder of a business empire that includes Virgin Atlantic Records and Virgin Airways. Having achieved enormous success in the business world, he still chooses pastimes full of acid-generating risk and excitement, such as skiing across ravines and attempting to circumnavigate the globe in a balloon.

At the local level, alkaline individuals can be found heading up community boards and spearheading fund-raising campaigns. I know women in these positions who have the energy to run a major corporation, often juggling their civic duties with a full-time career, managing a home and even raising a family at the same time. Our research assistant recounted a story about a friend of hers whose mother had had a stroke in her seventies. The grandmother, at age ninety-eight, stepped in to nurse her daughter. This is a feat that only an alkaline and unusually hearty oldster could do.

While few individuals have the alkaline constitution necessary to be president of the United States, secretary of state, or the CEO of their company, most of us would like to have, and in fact need, more physical energy and stamina to perform at an optimal level in our careers and in other areas of our lives. Unfortunately, as overacidity becomes a sad fact of life, usually between our thirties and sixties, fatigue, lack of stamina, and even physical exhaustion can occur. Overacidity can result from long hours of immobility spent working at one's desk or in front of a computer, overly acidic meals eaten hastily on the job, job-related stresses, and frequent travel. Luckily, we can once again enjoy a high level of physical energy as we improve our buffering capability and restore the body to its slightly alkaline pH.

The millions of overly acidic people in our society can improve their performance on the job and in their personal lives by restoring their buffering capability. This can be done through the use of a less acidic, more alkaline diet, alkaline minerals, and alkalinizing agents such as sodium and potassium bicarbonate (particularly helpful for prolonged periods of desk work and travel). Reducing one's level of stress and exposure to pollutants will also help to restore the body to a more healthful, slightly alkaline state.

Mental Clarity and Acuity

Individuals whose work requires intense mental activity and concentration will generate a great deal of acid in the process. Doing intellectual work for many hours at a time can greatly overburden the body's ability to buffer acids. This occurs, in part, because the brain consumes oxygen at a much faster rate when doing strenuous mental work, so reserves of this alkalinizing substance are diminished.

There is also a tendency during mental activities to take shallow breaths, so that less oxygen is inhaled and more acidic carbon dioxide is retained. People often become so involved in mental work that they will sit in a cramped position for hours without getting up to stretch or move around. This can result in the accumulation of acidic waste products in the tissues. After intense periods of mental work, most of us become tired as acidic wastes accumulate within the body. We may have to stop working for a short period of time until our pH balance has been restored and our mental energy returns.

High-alkaline producers, however, are able to do mental work for long periods of time without becoming fatigued. A good example of an individual with this trait was Margaret Thatcher, the former prime minister of Great Britain. While in office, she routinely needed little sleep, and she used her extra waking hours to study papers and reports in preparation for meetings. Even though her first appointment often took place as early as 6:00 a.m., she would be fully prepared to discuss the topics at hand with her advisors. Amazingly, she scheduled these meetings at fifteen-minute intervals. Such mental clarity is only possible in a person with an alkaline constitution.

If your job requires long periods of sitting at a desk or computer, it is important to take frequent, short, alkalinizing breaks away from your desk. Get up every 15-30 minutes to stretch or walk around your office or up and downstairs. Breathe deeply and slowly to begin to re-expand your lungs and re-oxygenate your body. Frequent breaks combined with physical activity will help reestablish your alkaline pH and allow you to maintain mental sharpness.

During particularly strenuous periods of mental exertion, make sure you are taking alkaline mineral supplements on a daily basis as well as one to five grams of mineral buffered vitamin C and one-half teaspoon of sodium bicarbonate or a sodium and potassium bicarbonate mixture (ranging from a 3:1 to a 4:1 ratio of sodium to potassium, depending on your tolerance for potassium) once or twice a day. Vitamin C (ascorbic acid) loses its natural acidity when buffered with alkaline minerals.

Preventing work-induced overacidity can help prevent job burnout. My natural tendency is to be overly acidic, but I take great care in restoring my own alkaline reserves to enable me to function as well as a naturally alkaline peak performer and write a lot of well thought through and researched books in a relatively short period of time each requiring intense mental work. If mental fatigue sets in, I just increase my alkalization by drinking a dosage of bicarbonate in water. Within a half-hour or so, my mental energy will be restored.

The Ability to Get Along With Other People

Many alkaline types channel their prodigious energy into socially beneficial activities. They are the leaders of their communities, businesses, and church groups. They are the organizers and doers. These individuals occupy the seats on the town councils and are the tireless fund-raisers who support every charitable cause that comes along. These people are intensely social, always at meetings, parties, and events.

In contrast, overly acidic individuals tend to lack the energy for intense social interactions and may even be withdrawn and introverted. The effect of pH on mental health is well demonstrated in the work of William H. Philpott, MD, an environmental psychiatrist who spent many years researching the links between food allergies, overacidity, and mood. In treating mental illness over a twenty-five-year period, he frequently observed that these conditions were often not emotional in origin but rather were due to chemical imbalances.

Dr. Philpott prescribed a combination of enzyme therapy and alkalinizing agents for patients who had severe psychological reactions to certain foods that they ate, and observed that their mental problems rapidly disappeared. Dr. Philpott described the case of a man who had suffered from autism as a child and schizophrenia in his teenage years. He discovered that this young man was severely overacidic. By restoring the patient to a normal alkaline pH through a variety of alkalinizing therapies, Dr. Philpott was able to get someone who had been fully dependent on his parents' care to drive a car and attend a university, where he studied art. The young man was eventually able to move out of his parents' house, live independently, and sell his artwork.

Optimism and Vision

There are many people who work in careers that require great optimism and vision. An example would be successful salespeople, who are able to envision the opportunity that they are offering a potential customer strongly enough for that person to see it, too—and then buy the product or service. To be successful, a salesperson must be able to sustain a positive outlook. In cold-call marketing, the difference between a salesperson who can't close deals and one who does is that the successful salesperson has the emotional stamina to keep making phone calls. Only an alkaline individual has the energy and tenacity required to maintain their optimism and enthusiasm in the face of frequent rejection.

Charitable fund-raisers also tend to be alkaline since they, too, need to maintain their enthusiasm and optimism in order to raise money for deserving causes. They must remain optimistic, with a can-do attitude, so that they can inspire people about the worthiness of the projects for which they are soliciting funds.

Artists, authors, and playwrights also have to maintain a positive frame of mind in order to gather their creative energies and produce works of art, often in the face of criticism and poor reviews if not outright rejection. Even if the statement an artist makes is full of doom and gloom, the very act of creating it requires an outgoing energy and the ability to stay focused on a goal. Overacidity can undermine creative work and silence the muses.

One physiological reason for the link between alkalinity and optimism is that overacidity acts as a depressant to the central nervous system, whereas alkalinity acts as a natural mood elevator. When acids accumulate in tissues throughout the body, they can directly affect the mental energy underlying our ability to create and maintain a positive outlook as much as our sex and stress hormones can affect mood.

Summary

A healthy alkaline balance enhances five important peak-performance traits, which shows how very important this function is in achieving success in all our endeavors.

4

Acid-Alkaline Imbalance and Health

Physicians normally deal with acid-alkaline related problems most often in hospitalized patients who have fluid and electrolyte imbalances. These imbalances are usually the result of the underlying disease process itself or occur as an undesirable side effect of medical therapy. As a result, much of the work done on acid-alkaline imbalances usually occurs on a crisis management basis. Many of these patients may have even lost their ability to buffer acid-alkaline imbalances adequately on their own.

However, the regulation of pH can be an important factor in the treatment of many diseases. This has been confirmed by hundreds of research studies. Once a decline in the efficiency of our pH-regulating system begins to occur, usually between our thirties and our sixties, many health problems begin to become more prevalent, in part because of overacidity. This is certainly the case with such common health issues such as the common cold, flus, sinusitis, bronchitis, middle-ear infections, allergies, and traumatic injuries.

Other common health issues such as digestive overacidity, bladder infections, kidney stones, rheumatoid arthritis, hypertension, and even cancer are also linked to overacidity. All of these conditions can be improved by restoring the body to its normal, slightly alkaline state.

Just as restoring alkalinity supports many peak-performance traits, it can also go a long way toward improving resistance to and preventing recurrences of many other common health conditions. These health conditions, in their turn, tend to compromise people's ability to perform at high levels in all aspects of their lives. Disease and chronic illness very understandably lead to absenteeism, reduced energy levels, and inability to perform job and personal responsibilities. Medical conditions of all kinds have a direct impact on peak performance, illustrating the interconnectedness of peak performance and overall health.

How Overacidity Affects Health

Many degenerative diseases are the result of the body becoming overly acidic. As mentioned earlier in this book, the cell, the basic unit of life, is alkaline. A healthy cell contains large amounts of alkaline substances like oxygen, bicarbonate, and alkaline minerals. All of our metabolic processes and the enzymes that initiate chemical reactions function their best in a slightly alkaline environment. However, the wear and tear of daily life and the aging process itself gradually cause our cells to lose their healthy alkalinity and become more acid over time, thereby making us more prone to disease. This can occur as a result of poor dietary habits, nutritional deficiencies, exposure to chemical pollutants, and emotional stress.

As mineral imbalances, a decrease in the level of oxygenation, and damage to our cells accumulate, the cells become too acidic. Depending on which tissues of the body become damaged and overly acidic, a variety of medical conditions can begin to develop. It is important to mention that the overacidity that occurs in many medical conditions is initially more of a localized phenomenon rather than a systemic problem, since the pH of the blood remains stable except in conditions of severe and even life-threatening illnesses. However, as health continues to decline with age, acidosis becomes more prevalent throughout the body. Thus acid-related conditions like digestive problems, allergies, gout, chronic fatigue, joint pains, and interstitial cystitis can coexist within the same individual. I describe some of these health conditions in this section.

Respiratory Illnesses

The most common health-related saboteurs in our society today are minor respiratory illnesses. When the body is overly acidic, a person is more susceptible to such ailments as colds, flus, bronchitis, sinusitis, and even pneumonia. The bacteria and viruses that cause these infections thrive in low-oxygen, acidic environments. Overacidity, due to a highly acidic diet, emotional stress, or poor oxygenation, makes a person more susceptible to respiratory infections.

The symptoms of respiratory illnesses—sneezing, sore throats, runny noses, and coughing—worsen as an individual becomes increasingly more acidic. In the more serious cases of respiratory infection, such as severe pneumonia, affected individuals can even develop respiratory acidosis, a potentially life-threatening condition in which the pH of the blood drops to dangerously low levels, and the lungs are no longer able to ventilate properly and make the necessary pH corrections by eliminating carbon dioxide from the body.

The statistics on the prevalence of respiratory ailments reflect how common overacidity is in the United States. The National Health Interview Survey estimated that there were 66 million cases of the common cold that resulted in either medical treatment or at least one day of restricted activity. This figure represents approximately 25 percent of the U.S. population. Given that most people do not go to a doctor when they develop a cold, the number of reported cases is all the more impressive. In the same year, 90 million people, or 45 percent of the population, were treated for the flu or had at least one day of downtime.

In addition, there were nearly 35 million cases of chronic sinusitis, 26 million cases of hay fever and allergy, 14 million cases of chronic bronchitis, and 14.5 million cases of asthma. Millions of children and adults suffer from middle-ear infections, which are triggered, in part, by overacidity due to allergy or sensitivity to dairy products. The prevalence of respiratory infections triggered by overacidity translates into an enormous drain on both individual and corporate resources as well as huge outlays of money spent on treating these conditions.

To counteract these ailments, Americans spend billions of dollars on over-the-counter remedies. Unfortunately, these products are relatively ineffective and have unpleasant side effects. They only provide symptom relief and do not help to restore the slightly alkaline pH of the body that is needed to recover rapidly from these conditions. Ironically, the medications themselves often increase acidity, retriggering the symptoms. No matter what medications respiratory illness sufferers use, recovery can be prolonged if the underlying overacidity of the system is not corrected.

Minor respiratory illnesses are health saboteurs because most people are often incapacitated by these episodes of colds, flus, bronchitis, and sinus infections. These conditions can persist for as long as one to six weeks, and many Americans, both adults and children, suffer from as many as four to six episodes each year. In fact, nasal conditions are one of the leading causes of lost productivity at school and work.

All of these conditions drastically reduce people's energy, create sleep disturbances, and impair concentration. They also greatly hamper socializing and make travel unpleasant. Their symptoms often occur at inopportune times and hinder consistent performance, causing sufferers to make uncharacteristic mistakes on the job, or even preventing them from showing up for work or social engagements. In addition, individuals with minor illnesses often feel miserable and tend to isolate themselves from coworkers, friends, and family members.

Traditional home remedies for colds and flus include drinking a glass of orange juice or ginger ale to settle the stomach, or eating a bowl of Jell-O.

While these might seem like comfort foods, they are highly acidic and will actually prolong recovery time. Instead, you should drink herbal teas (ginger tea is particularly good for the treatment of colds and flus) or vegetable or chicken broths. For the first twelve to twenty-four hours after the onset of symptoms, fasting on these liquids and avoiding solid food will help to bring the pH back into balance more rapidly. Remember, all food is eventually converted within the body to the acidic products of metabolism.

To rapidly suppress a respiratory infection, begin an alkalinization program immediately at the first sign of symptoms. Use one-half teaspoon of sodium bicarbonate (or sodium and potassium bicarbonate, taken in a 3:1 to a 4:1 ratio, depending on your tolerance for potassium.) Sodium bicarbonate may also be used alone if the mixture causes intestinal discomfort. Take the alkalinizing agent every one to two hours in the acute phase and then decrease to three to four times per day until the condition has been resolved for at least two days. Do not stop alkalinizing prematurely since the overacidic condition may not have been completely neutralized and symptoms may recur. You should also take one to three grams vitamin C buffered with alkaline minerals, taken in divided doses.

A Caution on Taking Bicarbonate of Soda

Very occasionally, a person will use too much bicarbonate and become overly alkaline. If this occurs, you may experience any of several symptoms, including a tingling sensation in the extremities, feeling overly energized, being unable to sleep, and, rarely, muscle spasms. If you should experience any of these symptoms, immediately discontinue use of the bicarbonate. Acidifying the system with a teaspoon or two of cider vinegar or the juice of half a lemon in water will help to neutralize the excess alkalinity.

You can try instituting treatment again the following day, but at a lower dosage and at less frequent intervals. If symptoms are severe, you may want to consult with your physician as to the advisability of using bicarbonate therapy at all for your particular case.

High-Alkaline Producers and Respiratory Illnesses

In contrast to the rest of us, individuals who are high-alkaline producers tend to be more resistant to respiratory illnesses. If they do come down with a cold or flu, overacidity is usually not the trigger. Often, other factors such as liver toxicity or diminished production of anti-inflammatory digestive enzymes or stress hormones may increase their susceptibility.

If these naturally alkaline individuals do come down with a cold or flu, they tend to recover quickly. They will leave work for a half day or a day, take a nap, eat lightly, and bounce right back. Interestingly, people with super functioning systems have no idea why they are this way. A good example of these disease-resistant types are physicians. Most family-practice doctors and pediatricians are exposed to respiratory infections from their patients on a regular basis. However, physicians tend to have hearty, alkaline constitutions—a prerequisite if a young doctor is to survive the rigors of the medical training process.

Occasionally, I see patients who have many of the signs of good buffering capability yet are poor oxygenators. This seemingly contradictory situation can occur in high-alkaline producers who have suffered lung damage, either due to environmental exposure or a prior lung infection. These individuals may maintain their naturally alkaline constitutions, yet they may still be prone to respiratory illnesses.

If you are a high-alkaline producer and develop a respiratory condition, then the old-fashioned remedy of orange juice and Jell-O is just what you need. Do not use alkalinizing agents since they will tend to overalkalinize you and will probably worsen your symptoms. Your condition is probably due to a chemical imbalance other than pH. In your case, the anti-inflammatory therapies, oxygen therapies, and detoxification therapies described in my other books would probably be most helpful in aborting a respiratory infection.

Two Success Stories

I want to share two stories of how my pH balancing program saved the day for both myself and my patient Roberta. Each of us has a story of how rapid treatment of respiratory infections with alkalinizing agents saved the day for us. The use of alkalinizing agents allowed us to resume our normal schedules very rapidly, despite the onset of severe respiratory symptoms. These infections would normally have caused us to be ill and functioning inefficiently for as long as two to three weeks.

Roberta's story. Since learning how to restore my acid-alkaline balance in my forties, I have been able to prevent the onset of or easily contain the symptoms of colds, flus, sinusitis, and bronchitis. These problems had plagued me since my early-childhood days. I am now able to eliminate these success saboteurs the way all naturally alkaline peak performers do. However, since I am not one of those individuals, I must always be ready to counter any tendency toward overacidity that can occur if I overstress my body beyond its normal pH tolerances. If you are like me and tend toward overacidity, the following story will show you the importance of always having a fully stocked alkalinizing kit available when traveling.

Several years ago, I scheduled a multicity cross-country trip, in mid-summer, to close a business deal that I had been working on for many months. Halfway into the scheduled ten-day trip, I realized it would have to be extended for at least another week. This meant more hotel living, airplane flights, and entertaining the potential business partners with rich foods and, often, too many cocktails and wine with dinner. The last city on the itinerary was New Orleans. Due to a shortage of rooms, I was given a room reserved for smokers (I have never smoked) that had been treated with toxic chemicals in an attempt to remove the smell of cigarette smoke. On top of that, the air conditioner's thermostat was set very low to combat the New Orleans summer heat and could not be adjusted by the hotel engineer.

The unhealthy conditions at the hotel plus the stress of travel, too much work, and all the rich food and drink sent me into a violently overacidic state. As I got on the plane to return to San Francisco, I knew I was coming down with something. Due to the length of the trip, I had used up my alkalinizing travel kit and sat on the six-hour flight without any emergency supplies. During the flight, I developed a sore throat, and my nose began to run. When I arrived home, I felt weak and was sneezing, coughing, and shaking with the chills, even though it was July. I immediately began an accelerated alkalinizing program, rested, and dramatically reduced my food intake. Within a few days, I was well on the road to recovery.

My Story. Several years ago, I pushed myself beyond my limits when I accepted numerous teaching engagements all over the state of California and was also completing several professional projects. I worked almost two months without a break, with relatively little sleep each night. Toward the end of the second month, I was driving to a weekend seminar where I was the featured lecturer. En route to the seminar, I stopped at a deli where I ate an extremely acidic meal consisting of salads and vegetables that seemed to be marinated in pure vinegar. The acidity of the meal coupled with my high level of work-related stress finally threw me into a state of extreme overacidity. As soon as I left the deli, I began to have a runny nose and couldn't stop sneezing. This occurred six hours before I was due to give my first lecture.

Fortunately, I had brought my buffering agents and supplements with me, as I usually do in case of an emergency. I started taking sodium and potassium bicarbonate every half hour for the first several hours, and then continued this regimen every hour. I also began to take digestive enzymes and buffered vitamin C to reduce the inflammation. After five hours of alkalinizing myself, I had restored my pH balance. My sneezing stopped, and the congestion cleared up almost entirely. I was able to meet my responsibilities and teach for the entire weekend, but I continued to use these alkalinizing agents to avoid a relapse.

Given how tired and stressed I was, there is no question that without these lifesavers I would have begun a downward spiral and spent a number of days in bed. By restoring my pH balance, however, I was able to get through a very busy weekend and continue with my normal schedule on Monday.

Business travel and lavish vacations create the perfect conditions for becoming overly acidic. Unless you are a high-alkaline producer, you should always take an emergency alkalinizing kit to ward off colds and flus when traveling for business or pleasure. The kit should contain an alkalinizing agent, buffered vitamin C, alkaline minerals, herbs such as ginger or curcumin with aspirin-like properties, and anti-inflammatory digestive enzymes.

Allergies and Sensitivities

Millions of Americans suffer from runny noses, sneezing, itching and tearing of the eyes, wheezing, abdominal pain, bloating, diarrhea, skin rash, and a propensity to middle-ear infections due to environmental or food allergies as well as food sensitivities. A wide variety of substances can trigger an allergic reaction, including pollens, molds, trees, and animal hairs as well as foods such as dairy products, wheat, corn, peanuts, and soy. Many individuals have sensitivities to foods such as wine, chocolate, tomatoes, oranges, and mushrooms as well as milk and fruit sugars either because of chemicals, such as amines, found in these foods or because they lack the enzymes needed to digest these foods.

The allergic response is triggered by mast cells. These are large cells found in connective tissue, particularly in the linings of the nose and lungs, as well as in the skin, the gastrointestinal tract, and reproductive organs. When an allergen is present, the mast cells release histamines and other chemicals that initiate the allergic response. This is actually the body's attempt to heal from the effects of the allergen. Histamines cause fluid to enter tissues of the affected areas, causing redness, swelling, and constriction of the smooth muscles.

The specific symptoms of an allergic reaction depend on where histamines are released. In the intestines, the result can be diarrhea. In the chest, histamines can cause coughing and asthma like symptoms (asthma is an extreme allergic reaction in which there is partial obstruction of the air passage to the lung as the muscles in these ducts contract). However, the severity of these symptoms depends on the degree of acidity of the internal environment.

When the body is overly acidic, and mast cells are activated by an allergen, they will tend to break down more quickly and are more likely to generate histamines and other inflammatory chemicals. Chronic inflammation can, in turn, damage cells and tissues, causing them to become even more acidic, thereby sending the body into a destructive downward spiral.

Overacidity can both trigger the symptoms of and lengthen the period of convalescence in allergic individuals. Unfortunately, the underlying cause is often overacidity, which is rarely treated. Obviously, environmental and food allergens and sensitizing agents should be avoided as much as possible. However, when a person is exposed to these substances, they should begin an aggressive alkalinizing program.

Allergic or sensitivity reactions can often be contained very quickly. Many people are unaware of the role that overacidity plays in their reactivity to allergens. Consider the following three cases:

Jonathan is a thirty-nine-year-old man who has suffered from allergies since childhood. With testing, he was found to be allergic to a wide variety of environmental allergens, including pollens, trees, and cat and dog hair. He was also sensitive to acid-forming foods such as dairy products and wheat, which his doctor had told him to avoid but which he ate anyway. His stressful job in finance also worsened his tendency toward overacidity.

Louise is a forty-eight-year-old woman who has suffered from recurrent episodes of bronchitis two or three times a year. These episodes were so disabling that she routinely missed a week to ten days of work each time she became ill. She was particularly prone to these episodes in the spring rainy season, when mold invaded her home. Allergy testing confirmed a mold allergy.

Laura is a fifteen-year-old high school sophomore with severe allergies to wheat, dairy products, and the milk and nuts contained within chocolate. Unfortunately, she had intense cravings for these foods, which she periodically binged on despite her mother's admonitions. These bingeing episodes were always followed by fatigue, sneezing, sore throats, and earaches, which caused her to be absent from school.

Avoiding the offending substances and following alkalinizing programs helped all of these individuals stop the downward cycle of allergic reactions that was undermining their health and well-being. Instituting a less acidic, more alkaline diet and using buffering agents and other supplements to reduce inflammation and build up their immunity has greatly improved their resistance to many allergens.

Traumatic Injury and Surgery

The use of alkalinizing agents can be helpful in healing any type of acute injury, whether traumatic or surgical. Any bodily injury will cause the injured tissue to become overly acidic. Individuals who are overly acidic and sustain a significant injury cause an added stress on their buffering capability. Injured tissue becomes relatively acidic because the swelling, hemorrhage, and other physical changes that occur within an injured area will impair oxygenation to these tissues. Diminished blood flow and the accumulation of waste products within the area also increase acidity. At the same time, there is an increase in metabolic activity and protein synthesis as the body's healing processes are activated.

The effect of injury on metabolism was discussed in a study published in the journal Muscle and Nerve. Volunteers who performed arm and leg exercises designed to cause mild muscle injury had elevated levels of inorganic phosphate in their muscle tissue for three to ten days. Since the processes of repair function best in an alkaline environment, supplementing with alkalinizing agents promotes healing within the injured area.

If you are overly acidic and tend to recover slowly from injuries, begin an alkalinizing program immediately following an acute injury. This should be done whether the injury is incurred taking part in strenuous physical activity or is due to trauma or surgery. Because injuries are always accompanied by inflammation, see my book on enzymes for the anti-inflammatory benefits of digestive enzymes and other supplements, if you are interested in this topic. Be sure to ask your physician about the advisability of following such a program if you have any specific questions.

Digestive Problems

Gastric overacidity is considered one of the most common digestive problems in the Western world. Pharmacies and supermarkets have shelves full of products designed to reduce the overacidity that occurs after a person has eaten something they cannot digest. Overacidity can stem from various causes. The stomach may secrete too much hydrochloric acid, even when there is no food in the stomach to be digested. At the same time, the pancreas may not be producing enough alkaline digestive juices to adequately buffer the acidic contents of the stomach as they move into the small intestines. When the pancreas produces insufficient amounts of bicarbonate, the enzymes necessary for digestion within the small intestines are unable to be activated.

Overacidity can also result from injury to the mucosa of the small intestine, leading to damage and acidosis of the underlying tissues. Crohn's disease, an inflammatory condition of the small intestine, or colitis due to acid stools can result from this overacidity. I see this problem frequently in midlife patients who suddenly find that they begin to have heartburn or digestive distress after eating highly acidic foods like pizza, steak, and orange juice.

However, heartburn may sometimes mask a more serious underlying condition. In a study done at the University of Oklahoma Medical Center, researchers assessed 178 patients with a long-term history of heartburn. Many of these patients reported using antacids for more than ten years. The study confirmed that almost all of them were sensitive to acid. However, over half also suffered from underlying conditions such as hiatus hernia (a condition in which stomach acid refluxes or backs up into the esophagus), and 40 percent suffered from an inflammatory condition called erosive esophagitis. Of greatest concern was that 7 percent were found to have serious underlying medical conditions like peptic ulcer disease, esophageal spasm, and cancer.

Sometimes people with symptoms of heartburn and gastric distress are actually producing too little hydrochloric acid in the stomach. Physicians practicing complementary medicine may find that patients who have weak pancreatic function (producing insufficient digestive enzymes and alkaline digestive juices) also produce insufficient amounts of stomach acid. These people tend to have poor digestive function at all levels of the digestive tract. They may suffer from food allergies as well as food intolerances. These individuals could actually benefit from hydrochloric acid supplementation to assist in the digestion of protein. Unfortunately, however, because of their poor buffering capability, they may be unable to tolerate the supplemental hydrochloric acid. In such individuals, hydrochloric acid capsules or drops may actually cause stomach burning and discomfort.

Some physicians find the use of Swedish bitters, artichoke bitters, and ginger tea to be effective substitutes for hydrochloric acid supplementation for patients who are both low acid producers in the stomach and low alkaline producers from the pancreas. (These individuals may also have reduced secretion of bile—which is also an alkalinizing substance needed to emulsify fats.) In addition, the amino acid glycine may also enhance gastric acid secretion (take 500 mg per day apart from meals).

Individuals with chronic, long-term symptoms of heartburn should have their symptoms evaluated by a physician to rule out a more serious condition.

Doctors usually recommend countering digestive overacidity with antacids or drugs that decrease the production of hydrochloric acid. Popular brands of antacids include Maalox, Mylanta, and Tums. These antacids tend to contain various types of alkaline mineral substances such as magnesium oxide or hydroxide, aluminum hydroxide, magnesium trisilicate, and calcium carbonate.

Alka-Seltzer is another short-term remedy for indigestion used by millions of people. This product is simply sodium bicarbonate combined with citric acid. When water is added to this mixture, an effervescent gas is released, turning the Alka-Seltzer powder into a bubbling drink.

Both calcium citrate and sodium citrate are also useful as buffering agents for counteracting digestive overacidity. A study published in the South African Medical Journal found that in thirty healthy volunteers, a sodium citrate preparation raised the pH level of the stomach significantly. The researchers measured gastric acid output after a single 12 g dose and found that the stomach pH rose to 3.0. (The stomach normally has a pH of 1.5 to 2.5.) Similar results were achieved after three to six days of continuous therapy, using 4 g and 12 g dosages. In addition, calcium citrate has been shown to be an effective antacid for patients with kidney disease who can no longer regulate their pH effectively.

The alternative to the above remedies is to take a medication that suppresses acid production completely. Many foods and caffeine stimulate receptors within the stomach to secrete stomach acid, and a class of drugs has been developed to block this action. Many are sold without prescription, such as Zantac, Pepcid, Axid, and Tagamet. All these treatments are meant to reduce the annoying symptoms of overacidity such as gas, bloating, nausea, constipation, and diarrhea.

Although taking antacids can be very effective in relieving digestive symptoms, the timing of their use is very important. If antacids are taken with meals, or right after eating, they can interfere with the digestion of food. Antacids neutralize the hydrochloric acid produced by the stomach, which in turn inactivates the enzymes that are essential for the breakdown of protein.

This makes it difficult for the body to effectively digest foods such as meat, milk, wheat, and nuts and beans (all of which contain hard-to-digest protein), and to efficiently extract the minerals that these foods contain.

A Caution on Using Antacids

In rare cases, the use of antacids can also lead to systemic alkalosis, raising pH throughout the body. Symptoms of alkalosis include tingling in the lips or extremities, tense muscles, anxiety, or an unusually strong surge of energy after taking an alkalinizing agent. If you experience these symptoms, stop taking the antacid, and restart at a much smaller dose taken at greater intervals. If symptoms are severe, you may want to consult with your physician as to the advisability of using antacids. The next chapter provides more specific information on how to best use these various products to counteract overacidity.

It is helpful to wait one to one and one-half hours after a heavy protein meal before taking the antacid. Some people, however, produce such large amounts of acid that they begin to feel discomfort immediately upon eating. These people may need to use antacids with the meal.

Cystitis or Bladder Infections

Several research studies confirm the usefulness of alkalinizing therapies for cystitis, an inflammatory condition of the bladder caused by bacterial infection. Cystitis is a very common ailment, with millions of cases being treated by physicians each year. Women tend to be infected more readily than men, due to their short urethra, which allows for easier bacterial contamination of the bladder. While cystitis can occur in women of all ages, it is particularly prevalent in postmenopausal women, due to age-related changes in which the walls of the urethra thin out and become drier. It is estimated that 10 to 15 percent of women over age sixty have frequent bladder infections.

Bacteria can thrive and multiply in the warm, wet urine within the bladder. As the bacteria attack the lining of the bladder, superficial erosion of the lining can occur, which exposes this sensitive tissue to the irritating effects of urine. Individuals with cystitis frequently experience a burning sensation or a feeling of pressure in the bladder area, as well as the need to urinate frequently.

Antibiotics are prescribed as the usual treatment for this condition. However, with the increasing resistance of the bacteria causing these infections to a number of antibiotics, alternative therapies may be quite helpful in eradicating infection and reducing symptoms. Drinking cranberry juice, which acts as an acidifying agent, has traditionally been recommended as a home treatment under the rationale that chemicals contained in cranberries prevent the bacteria within the bladder from adhering to its lining. However, the form of cranberry juice readily available in the supermarket is loaded with sugar because the pure juice is so tart. By adding sugar to the bladder, the juice may actually promote the growth of bacteria. In addition, the pure juice is so acidic that it is best used only by high-alkaline producers.

In contrast, both the clinical experience of some physicians and several research studies support the use of two alkalinizing agents, sodium citrate and potassium citrate, for the treatment of bladder infections. The use of alkalinizing agents may actually be more useful for overly acidic individuals who tend to have bladder infections. Because potassium citrate tends to be unpalatable, the much blander sodium citrate preparations are preferable.

In a study published in the Journal of International Medical Research, 205 women between the ages of eighteen and sixty with typical symptoms of cystitis, but only 20 percent of whom showed large amounts of bacteria in the urine, were treated with sodium citrate. (This is not unusual since clinical symptoms and urine culture results do not always correlate well.) Each volunteer was asked to take 4 g of sodium citrate in a glass of water three times a day for forty-eight hours (4 g is equal to 1/7 oz.). At the conclusion of the treatment period, 80 percent of the women without bacteria in their urine reported significant relief of symptoms; about 50 percent of the women whose initial urine cultures showed evidence of a bacterial infection also experienced symptom relief as well as a clearing of the urine.

In a further study, sixty-four women were also given sodium citrate every eight hours for two days. Eighty percent of these women noted relief of their symptoms, while 12 percent found that their symptoms became worse. These results were similar to the earlier study in that women with symptoms but no evidence of bacteria in the urine had more uniform results than those women with proven bacterial infections. A study published in the European Journal of Microbiology and Infectious Disease found that alkalinizing the urine improved the ability of the body to destroy and eliminate the bacteria.

The following simple steps will help both to eradicate bladder infections and to prevent their recurrence: (1) Take 5 to 10 g of buffered vitamin C each day (that's 5000 to 10,000 mg), divided into four dosages; and (2) avoid acidic foods such as coffee, soft drinks, sugar, and alcoholic beverages.

Interstitial Cystitis

Interstitial cystitis is another type of bladder disease; it is frequently mistaken for bacterial cystitis. This condition occurs when there is inflammation between the bladder lining and the bladder muscles. This is a chronic condition that can be far more painful and debilitating than ordinary bacterial cystitis. While the great majority of patients are women, men sometimes develop this ailment.

Interstitial cystitis occurs when the lining of the bladder becomes chronically irritated. The frequent use of antibiotics, hormones, exposure to viruses, and a history of prior bladder infections can damage the bladder lining and increase the risk of developing this condition. In a healthy bladder, the tissues lining it secrete a mucus-like substance that forms a protective barrier. This barrier consists of sugar, an amino acid, and sulfur, and is called the GAG layer. The GAG layer protects the underlying tissue from being colonized by bacteria. It also helps to maintain the integrity of the bladder lining, which is constantly exposed to acidic urine, food, pollutants, and chemicals. If the protective GAG layer is damaged or destroyed, the cells of the bladder can become damaged. As a result, the cells begin to lose their normal state of healthy alkalinity as they lose bicarbonate. At the same time, they gain hydrogen ions (protons), causing them to become more acidic.

In the early stages of the disease, when urine begins to erode through the tissues of the bladder lining, individuals affected will experience a feeling of urgency to urinate. With further erosion of the GAG layer, these symptoms begin to worsen as the bladder becomes scarred and ulcerated. There may be a nearly constant sensation of pressure and burning in the bladder, pain during intercourse, and fatigue, as well as such diverse symptoms as sore throat, headache, diarrhea, bowel problems, joint pains, and asthma like symptoms. The bladder may also shrink to hold only one or two ounces of urine.

The consumption of acidic foods can immediately trigger symptoms. Patients with interstitial cystitis frequently complain of pain and burning after ingesting foods with an acidic pH or foods that are highly acid-forming or inflammatory, like citrus fruits and juices, chocolate, spicy foods, coffee, black tea, soft drinks, and alcoholic beverages. Acidic vitamin C (ascorbic acid) also increases symptoms. Painful symptoms can occur almost immediately after ingesting the offending food or substance. Symptoms can also be triggered by emotional stress.

To test for interstitial cystitis, a urine sample is normally analyzed for the presence of bacteria. The urine should show no sign of bacterial infection and often has an alkaline pH. As mentioned above, when bladder cells are damaged, they become more acidic. They leak their contents into the urine, losing their alkaline minerals while, at the same time, gaining acidic hydrogen ions from the surrounding environment. Thus the cells become more acidic while the urine pH begins to rise. The overacidity of the cells makes it more difficult for the bladder tissue to repair itself.

Several alkalinizing agents can be very useful in treating interstitial cystitis. Sodium bicarbonate can provide almost instantaneous relief of symptoms by helping the bladder tissue become more alkaline. Calcium carbonate or sodium citrate can be taken several times per day to slowly release bicarbonate into the bladder tissues (sodium citrate has been found to partially convert to carbonate within the bladder). Anti-inflammatory agents such as digestive enzymes and MSM (methylsulfonylmethane) are also helpful in treating interstitial cystitis.

Kidney Stones

Kidney stones are very common in our society, affecting about 10 percent of the population. They occur more frequently in men than women. The recurrence rate is high, with 20 to 50 percent of the individuals affected forming new stones. Kidney stones are also an expensive problem to treat, with $2 billion spent annually on medical therapy.

Five to 10 percent of them are uric-acid stones. Individuals with gout or who have an elevated uric-acid level in the blood are at higher risk of forming these stones. Alkalinizing the urine helps to make the uric acid more soluble so that stones are less likely to form. Alkalinizing agents such as sodium and potassium citrate are also used in the treatment of kidney stones, both to dissolve the stones and to prevent their recurrence.

One study, published in Drug Intelligence and Clinical Pharmacology, reported that fifty-three patients with uric-acid stones who were treated with potassium citrate had a reduction in the number of stones formed and less likelihood of recurrence. During the period of treatment, which lasted from one to one and one-half years, between 75 and 92 percent of the patients went into remission.

Individuals who tend to form uric-acid kidney stones should limit their intake of foods such as meat that contain purines, which convert to uric acid as they are metabolized. Instead they should follow a more vegetarian-based, less acid, more alkaline diet. Vitamin C should be taken in a buffered form rather than as ascorbic acid. Aspirin, another acidic compound, should be avoided. Drinking plenty of water on a daily basis is also recommended to help maintain a dilute urine.

Magnesium has also been added to preparations of potassium citrate. This combination has been found to be very effective in reducing the recurrence of stones. Researchers at a Kaiser Permanente Medical Care Program in Oakland, California, gave this compound to sixty-four patients who had a tendency to form kidney stones on a recurrent basis, over a three-year period. According to their study, published in the Journal of Urology, the researchers found that while untreated patients had a 69 percent recurrence rate, only 13 percent of those receiving the magnesium and potassium citrate subsequently developed kidney stones. Another benefit to adding magnesium to this regimen was that it reduced the unpalatability of the potassium citrate.

Rheumatoid Arthritis and Other Autoimmune Diseases

Rheumatoid arthritis is a disabling and crippling inflammatory disease of the joints. It chiefly affects the synovial membrane (a thick tissue covering the joints) of the small joints of the body. Symptoms include joint stiffness, especially in the morning, tenderness, warmth, and pain, most often in the joints of the fingers, wrists, toes, ankles, and knees. Other symptoms include fever, fatigue, loss of appetite and weight, and depression. As the disease progresses, the joints thin out and become deformed. Cartilage, bone, ligaments, and tendons in and around the joints are weakened or destroyed, which can lead to muscle atrophy and imbalances of opposing groups of muscles.

While rheumatoid arthritis can occur anytime in life, 70 percent of the cases are diagnosed between the ages of thirty and seventy with the peak incidence in the fourth decade. It is estimated that approximately 10 percent of all people sixty-five years of age and older suffer from this condition. Women with this disease outnumber men by a ratio of almost 3:1.

Many research studies have implicated diet as a major risk factor in the development of rheumatoid arthritis. All of the foods that have been found to worsen the symptoms of this disease are either highly acidic or produce an acid response within the body. When volunteers with this disease were taken off these foods and either fasted for a period of time or were placed on more alkaline vegetarian diets, they experienced a notable improvement in their symptoms. One such study, published in Clinical Allergy, placed twenty-two patients on an elimination diet in which highly acidic and allergenic foods were excluded from their daily intake. Twenty out of the twenty-two patients noted an improvement in their symptoms.

In another study, published in the Scandinavian Journal of Rheumatology, twenty-seven patients with rheumatoid arthritis were taken off their customary highly acidic diet, fasted for seven to ten days, and were then placed sequentially on a wheat-free vegan diet for three and one-half months followed by a lacto-vegetarian diet for nine months. Twenty-six rheumatoid sufferers in a control group continued to eat their normal, highly acidic, meat-based diet. Twelve of the twenty-seven patients on the more alkaline vegetarian diet noted an improvement in their symptoms, whereas only two people in the control group noted similar relief during the study period.

Although vegetarian diets have been found to promote symptom relief in individuals with rheumatoid arthritis, including fish in the diet also appears to be beneficial. This is because the polyunsaturated fatty acids contained in fish like salmon, tuna, trout, and halibut are converted within the body to very potent, hormone-like, anti-inflammatory chemicals called series III prostaglandins. Several studies, including a study published in Clinical Allergy, a study published in Lancet, and a study published in the Annals of the Rheumatic Diseases, found that fish-based diets reduced morning stiffness and the number of tender joints that volunteers complained of as well as laboratory indicators of inflammation. In contrast, volunteers who ate diets high in saturated fats had no improvement in their symptoms.

A study published in the American Journal of Clinical Nutrition suggested that flax seed oil, another series III prostaglandin precursor, could be substituted for fish oil as a potent anti-inflammatory substance. Thus, fish and flax seed oil decrease the production of highly acidic inflammatory chemicals within the body, which can greatly benefit arthritis sufferers. I have found one to two tablespoons of flax seed oil to be highly effective in treating her arthritis patients.

Rheumatoid arthritis is a significant problem for people who work with their hands, such as computer programmers, physical therapists, people involved in assembly work, illustrators, and artists. Because these individuals are involved in precision work, this disease can significantly affect their ability to earn a living. I have treated many such patients. In most cases, my patients ate a very acidic diet and were unaware of the effect that their food choices were having on their disease. Many of these individuals improved significantly after modifying their eating habits, using alkalinizing agents, and following a number of other therapies described in this book. The following case exemplifies the usefulness of an alkalinizing program.

Dorothy is a fifty-one-year-old executive secretary whose work requires that she spend many hours a day doing word processing on a computer. When she first consulted me, she was suffering from severe pain and stiffness in her fingers. Upon examination, I found that Dorothy's joints were already moderately deformed and swollen. After taking a dietary history, I found that Dorothy's favorite foods, such as red meat, wheat pasta, dairy products, and sugary desserts, were highly acidic or acid forming. Dorothy was initially unhappy at the idea of giving up so many of her preferred foods but was highly motivated to do anything that would reduce her symptoms.

As a self-supporting single woman, she did not relish the idea of quitting an excellent job that she truly enjoyed. She made a number of dietary changes over a three-month period, eliminating the highly acidic foods from her diet and finding more alkaline substitutions that satisfied her tastes. She also started an alkalinizing program as well as a strong program of nutritional supplements designed to help support and rebuild her joints. She made steady progress during this period and was pleased to report significant decreases in her joint stiffness and discomfort.

Besides rheumatoid arthritis, many other autoimmune diseases—such as thyroiditis, Crohn's disease, colitis, and systemic lupus erythematosus—are worsened by highly acidic diets. A less acidic, more alkaline diet should be used by individuals suffering from any of these conditions.

Besides taking alkalinizing agents and eating a more alkaline diet, you may find that anti-inflammatory supplements such as digestive enzymes, curcumin, and MSM (methylsulfonylmethane) can be very useful in the treatment of arthritis and other inflammatory conditions. See my book on enzymes for more information on these remedies.

Gout

While not as prevalent as rheumatoid arthritis, gout is another disabling joint disease. Gout occurs when there is an excess of uric acid in the blood, causing crystals of uric acid to be deposited in the tissues surrounding the joints. Gout can affect many different joints, including the big toe. (Prints done in the eighteenth century often portray gout suffers sitting in large, overstuffed chairs, with their red and throbbing foot propped on a hassock.)

Acute attacks of gout are particularly painful, causing severe, viselike pain that can last for two to ten days. Attacks will often occur early in the morning upon awakening if a person has eaten a dinner of highly acidic foods, such as meat and alcohol, the night before. Symptoms of gout may also occur after surgery and as a side effect of taking certain medications. As men age, they are more likely to have gout than women, but after menopause, the risk for females increases also.

Gout is linked to high levels of purines produced by the body and consumed in the diet. Purines are found in foods such as red meat, whole grains, and legumes. The body converts purines to uric acid, which circulates in the blood. The uric acid is then excreted in the urine or via the digestive tract. Individuals with gout should avoid highly acidic foods and instead eat a more alkaline, vegetarian-based diet.

Since individuals with gout are more likely to form uric-acid stones than the rest of the population, the use of alkalinizing agents may also be helpful in individuals who have both conditions.

Osteoporosis

Osteoporosis is one of the most common diseases of old age. It occurs when the bones lose their alkaline mineral reserves and become thin, porous, and progressively weaker. Osteoporosis is most prevalent among postmenopausal women, affecting nearly one-third of all women. The incidence of fractures of the hip, wrist, and spine due to osteoporosis increases significantly by the sixth and seventh decades. About 10 to 15 percent of all men also develop osteoporosis.

While doctors normally treat osteoporosis with hormone replacement therapy, vitamin D, and calcium supplements, they often do not address the underlying overacidity that causes the demineralization of the bone. The bones contain one of our major reserves of alkaline minerals such as calcium. Ninety-nine percent of the calcium in our bodies is in the bones. If the body becomes overly acidic, and the other buffer systems are inadequate, calcium and other alkaline minerals are released from the bones to keep the pH of the blood stable.

Any successful treatment of osteoporosis should address the acidity of the diet. One of the major sources of acid in the diet is meat. Not only is meat high in acid, but its tough fibrous protein causes the stomach to secrete large amounts of hydrochloric acid, which is necessary to begin the breakdown of this protein into its constituent amino acids. Processed foods also contain many phosphate food additives.

Coffee is another highly acidic substance that is widely consumed in our culture. According to a study published in the American Journal of Clinical

Nutrition, women with calcium intake lower than 750 mg a day who drink more than two or three cups of coffee on a daily basis showed an increased loss of bone mass.

Another study, published in the American Journal of Clinical Nutrition, found that an increase in protein intake from 44 g to 102 g resulted in a significant increase in the urinary excretion of calcium and a lowering of the pH of the urine. Treatment with a small amount of sodium bicarbonate reversed this effect by alkalinizing the urine and reducing calcium excretion.

Researchers also compared the effect of a meat-based diet to that of a lacto-vegetarian diet on bone mass in elderly white women. Interestingly, they found that a diet high in animal protein led to more loss of bone mass than a vegetarian diet, even if both diets provided ample protein. Their study, which was published in the Journal of the American Dietetic Association, found that women who followed a lacto-vegetarian diet had an 18 percent decrease in their bone mass, while the women who included meat in their diet lost 35 percent of their bone mass, nearly double that of the other group.

While a less acid, more alkaline diet slows the loss of bone mass in postmenopausal women, adding a buffering agent to the treatment program can significantly reduce bone demineralization. An interesting study documenting the benefits of potassium bicarbonate was published in the New England Journal of Medicine. Eighteen healthy postmenopausal women were given potassium bicarbonate coupled with a diet that provided 80 g of protein per day, an amount typically found in the standard American diet. Potassium bicarbonate therapy reduced the excretion of both acid and calcium in the urine. It also promoted new bone growth and caused a decrease in bone loss. A separate study, using sodium bicarbonate, found that alkalinization reduced calcium loss and improved calcium balance within the body.

Diabetes

In insulin-dependent diabetes, the pancreas no longer produces sufficient insulin. (Insulin is the hormone that allows sugar or glucose to be transported across the cell membrane so that it can be used by the cell as its major source of energy.) As a result, glucose levels rise in the blood after ingesting a meal. Elevated blood sugar levels can have an acidifying effect on the blood and the tissues throughout the body, since sugar is acidic.

Many treatments to reduce the stress on the pancreas include using insulin as a replacement therapy and taking nutritional supplements such as chromium, manganese, zinc, B vitamins, and digestive enzymes to facilitate glucose metabolism. In insulin-dependent diabetes, pancreatic production of alkalinizing bicarbonate may also be impaired. In such cases, eating a less acidic, more alkaline diet that emphasizes vegetables, fruits such as papayas and melons, and certain grains and legumes is also highly recommended.

Hypertension

Hypertension, or high blood pressure, is a condition in which the blood pressure is elevated above 140/90 mm Hg. In this condition, the muscular layer of the blood vessels constricts. There may also be an accumulation of plaque on the walls of the blood vessels. As a result, the passageway through which the blood must flow narrows. The heart must then pump harder to circulate blood to the tissues. Approximately 60 percent of Americans over the age of sixty have high blood pressure. African Americans, people who are overweight, diabetics, or individuals who have a family history of high blood pressure are more likely to develop this condition. Hypertension increases the risk of heart attacks and strokes as well as kidney and eye problems.

Various medications have proven effective in the treatment of high blood pressure. However, all medications have negative side effects such as loss of essential minerals, impotence, or elevation of the blood sugar level. Many people are able to manage mild to moderate high blood pressure simply through lifestyle changes. These include weight loss, following a low-fat and low-salt diet, and stress reduction techniques such as biofeedback.

Alkalinizing the body can also reduce high blood pressure. For many years, the standard treatment was the use of potassium chloride. However, recent studies suggest that the acidic chloride component of this compound may actually raise blood pressure. In an animal study, Dr. Curtis Morris and his colleagues at the University of California, San Francisco, compared the effect of different salts on blood pressure. They tested table salt (sodium chloride), potassium chloride, and two nonchloride, alkaline forms of salts found in plants, potassium bicarbonate and potassium citrate.

The researchers found that potassium bicarbonate and potassium citrate actually lowered blood pressure and reduced the incidence of stroke. Their work also suggested that the chloride in table salt or combined with other minerals as a salt may trigger high blood pressure.

Cancer

Many factors are known to increase the risk of cancer in susceptible individuals. These include genetic factors, familial predisposition, dietary factors, and exposure to toxic chemicals. Some studies have also suggested that an acidic cellular environment seems to be a predisposing factor for the development of certain cancers. This connection was first discussed in a landmark paper by Otto Warburg, MD, who received two Nobel prizes for his work. His paper, entitled "On the Origin of Cancer Cells," was published in 1952 in the journal Science. Dr. Warburg was the first to propose that a deficiency of oxygen (a highly alkaline element) within the cells caused changes in the cellular metabolism leading to the development of cancer.

Dr. Warburg found that normal, healthy cells depend on an adequate supply of oxygen along with glucose (sugar) for the production of their energy needs. When deprived of oxygen, cells revert to a more primitive, fermentative metabolism, which is typical of cancer cells as well as disease-causing bacteria and fungi. The end product of fermentation is lactic acid, a substance that causes cells to have a lower pH. The amount of energy that can be produced by fermentation is eighteen times less than the amount that can be optimally produced by cells that are well oxygenated. The lack of oxygen thereby limits the amount of energy available to the cell to carry out its normal metabolic functions.

Although Dr. Warburg's original work has been modified by subsequent research, many studies have found that certain types of cancers can be treated effectively with oxygen therapies, because of their alkalinizing and tumor-destroying effects, as well as a less acidic, more alkaline diet. Oxygen therapies are discussed in detail in my book on oxygen therapies. Many other factors thought to promote cancer also produce overacidity within the body. These include free radicals, food allergies, aberrant electromagnetic energy, industrial chemicals, and other environmental toxins.

However, highly alkaline individuals who develop cancer should not be treated with alkalinizing agents since they can create severe imbalances in these individuals. Other types of cancer treatments, such as enzyme and detoxification therapies and many other treatment options, would be more appropriate and more beneficial, depending on the type of tumor.

High-Alkaline Producers and Health

While individuals who are high-alkaline producers represent only a small fraction of the population, their strong constitutions provide them with remarkable resistance to disease. They often have great reservoirs of alkaline minerals contained within their cells, tissues, and bones that give them ample buffering capability well into old age. Even in their eighties and nineties, they do not tend to develop many of the common diseases related to overacidity, such as osteoporosis, kidney, or lung failure—provided, of course, that their other physiological functions remain strong.

High-alkaline producers need to constantly create acid within their bodies to stay in balance, through a highly acidic diet, physical exertion, and a fast-paced, busy life. While naturally alkaline individuals thrive on the types of diets, activities, and stresses that are toxic to almost everyone else, the converse is also true: They need to avoid the types of lifestyle choices that are most beneficial to their more acidic peers. For example, their dietary needs run counter to the current recommendation of a less acidic, more alkaline, vegetarian-based regimen espoused by Dean Ornish, MD, the Longevity Center, and even the American Cancer Society.

When these people do try to follow the trends and adopt a low-fat, low-protein, and high-complex carbohydrate diet with a more vegetarian emphasis on grains and starches as well as fruits and vegetables, they feel weak, devitalized, and mentally foggy. Eating this way will cause them to lose their natural robust energy and stamina, and their performance in many areas will begin to suffer. Some of my patients who are high-alkaline producers have felt terrible when they have tried to eliminate meat from their diet. Naturally alkaline people instinctively gravitate to a highly acidic diet of red meat, soft drinks, sugar, white-flour products, beer, wine, caffeinated beverages, and fruit juices in order to maintain their pH within the normal range.

A patient that I saw exemplifies this issue. Alex was a forty-seven-year-old businessman who was raised in an eastern European family. His family continued to eat their traditional diet, which was high in meat protein and saturated fat, long after they resettled in the United States. Alex continued to eat this way throughout his entire adult life. A physically strong and highly energetic individual, he was concerned about his elevated cholesterol level because of a strong family history of heart disease. After reading several books on cardiovascular health, he tried to become a vegetarian. After a week of eating mostly grains, yams, beans, raw salads, and steamed vegetables, he no longer felt like himself and complained of feeling tired and listless. He quickly went back to his old dietary habits until I revised his diet toward a more healthy lean meat, vegetable, and omega 3 fatty acid emphasis regimen.

While alkaline individuals are not prone to diseases related to overacidity, they may have a higher risk of heart attacks, strokes, and cancer of the prostate and colon than their peers who follow a more vegetarian-based diet. Since the digestive function of most high-alkaline producers is so strong, they typically eat a diet high in animal protein and saturated fat. This may result in elevated blood lipids and the buildup of plaque within the arteries, thereby increasing their risk of cardiovascular disease. This is a common scenario among hard-driving, typically alkaline CEOs, who run their companies with enormous energy and staying power right up to the time that they have their first heart attack, in their fifties or sixties.

Although many of these individuals need the acidity of meat to remain healthy, they would do better to eliminate red meat and dairy products and eat fish instead. For while fish provides needed protein, it also provides healthy polyunsaturated oils, which lower cholesterol, prevent clotting, and promote cardiovascular health. However, I should clarify that although these individuals can handle the acidity of the standard American diet, this diet in no way provides the essential nutrients that all individuals, whether naturally alkaline or overly acidic, need to maintain their health and well-being.

High-alkaline producers are better served by following a diet that is both highly acidic and nutrient rich. This type of diet includes seafood, poultry, vegetables, fruits, legumes, whole grains, and condiments like vinegar—basically, a more highly acidic version of the Mediterranean diet. However, while naturally alkaline people can eat more of the meat, fruit, and vinegar-doused pasta, vegetables, and salads, overly acidic people should emphasize more of the vegetables, whole grains, and legumes of this regimen. In addition, these individuals should significantly decrease their intake of highly acidic foods and beverages that have a deleterious effect on health. This category includes alcohol, coffee, tea, soft drinks, and rich, sugary desserts.

On my recommendation, Joseph began to substitute omega 3 rich fish and free-range poultry for the fatty red meat that was his chief source of protein and significantly increased his intake of a wide variety of vegetables. He also began to supplement his diet with various types of fiber to help promote the elimination of cholesterol from his body. Within six months, his cholesterol level had dropped significantly.

The fatty foods that alkaline types tend to eat can also lead to weight gain. This is particularly true if these individuals are older and have begun to lose their oxygenating ability. As oxygen intake begins to decline, people burn calories less efficiently. Since fat has more than twice the number of calories of protein and starch, eating a high-fat diet can easily lead to weight gain. It is very common in our country to see a stockily built, physically strong middle-aged man with a noticeable belly. To counteract this tendency, alkaline individuals need to reduce their fat intake by eating leaner cuts of meat, more salads and steamed vegetables, and the healthier fats and oils, such as extra-virgin olive oil, rather than butter.

Naturally alkaline peak performers also have a need for constant excitement, activity, hard physical exertion, and even stress, which runs counter to the current advice promoting the health benefits of stress management and a relaxed and moderate lifestyle. Remember, these people are continually producing large amounts of alkaline buffers, so they need to generate acid through their lifestyles to stay within a normal pH range.

Finally, these individuals should avoid antacids such as baking soda (sodium bicarbonate) and Tums. Although these remedies help tens of millions of Americans counter the ill effects of gastric overacidity, canker sores, and other minor ailments related to overacidity, I have seen them produce toxic effects in her naturally alkaline patients. These people tend to become bloated, gassy, fatigued, and even panicky when using these remedies since they tend to push these individuals' pH even further toward the alkaline side (of course, overly acidic individuals should avoid the overuse of antacids also).

Finally, severe diarrhea can cause the body to lose a significant amount of acid minerals in a short period of time, thereby causing overalkalinity in anyone, of either acid or alkaline constitution. This type of diarrhea is often associated with eating contaminated foods either while camping, eating at a restaurant or social gathering, or visiting a foreign country. To resolve this condition and restore a normal pH balance, drink a sugar and salt solution, which will replace the lost electrolytes, including the acid minerals. These solutions are readily available in pharmacies and health food stores. If you do a lot of camping, you may wish to keep some electrolyte solutions at your base camp.

Summary

Overacidity affects health in a wide variety of ways, from digestive problems, infectious diseases, and arthritis to such diseases as high blood pressure, osteoporosis, and cancer. Fortunately, each condition can be treated to some extent by correcting the acid-alkaline balance of the body through a combination of dietary changes and the use of alkalinizing agents.

5

Testing for Acid-Alkaline Balance

There are several methods to assess your acid-alkaline balance including both self-testing and laboratory testing. I discuss them both in this chapter. While none of these tests are definitive, they can still be helpful indicators in understanding your acid-alkaline status.

Self-Testing for Acid-Alkaline Balance

A pH test of your saliva or urine may be used in addition to the checklists to help assess your relative acidity or alkalinity. You can buy pH Hydrion test paper at your local pharmacy and use it to test the acidity of your saliva or urine. This product consists of a roll of pH paper to test your body fluids and a color-graded pH chart. When the pH test paper is saturated with saliva or urine, it develops a color. The paper is then held next to the color chart to find the matching color, which indicates the pH. The spectrum of colors moves from yellow (acid) to dark blue (alkaline). Inexpensive pH meters are also available commercially and can be used to test body fluids as well as water and beverages.

While any particular spot test of the pH of your saliva or urine is not particularly helpful, measuring them periodically over a six- to twelve-month period may help you assess the effectiveness of an alkalinizing program. To assess the pH of your saliva, a saliva sample should be taken one hour either before or after a meal. An average saliva pH can be obtained by taking a sample twice a day, at the same times, for seven days. This will give fourteen values, which are added and then divided by 14 to give an average reading. This series of tests can then be repeated in four to six weeks. The normal pH of the saliva is 6.0 to 7.5, which is needed to begin the digestion of starches in the mouth. To assess the pH of your urine, sample the first urine you void in the morning.

However, pH tests of urine and saliva need to be interpreted cautiously and only in concert with other medical testing and your medical history. This is because these tests do not simply reflect your internal acid-alkaline milieu but can also vary greatly in response to changes in your diet, levels of stress and exercise, and even exposure to environmental toxins. For example, a highly acidic meal, a stressful situation, or vigorous physical exertion can cause a rapid acidification of the body, which must be immediately corrected through the buffer systems which were previously described. In contrast, the excessive use of alkalinizing agents also has to be corrected through these buffer systems. These fluctuations can cause shifts in the pH of the saliva and urine. My dentist has routinely tested the pH of his patients' saliva to help him determine the appropriate type of filling material to use.

There is another very simple indicator that will give you an idea of whether you tend to be overly acidic or are a high-alkaline producer. Overly acidic people will tend to feel better and have more energy when they take one-half - one teaspoon each day of sodium bicarbonate (baking soda). They will not feel as well or develop digestion symptoms when they eat more acidic foods like vinegar or caffeinated beverages like soft drinks or coffee. In contrast, however, high-alkaline producers are normally able to tolerate highly acidic foods like vinegar, lemon juice or carbonated soft drinks without ill effect, while overly acidic people may find that eating these same foods causes canker sores, heartburn, bladder pain, or sore throats, to name but a few symptoms.

People with healthy, well-balanced buffering capabilities can usually tolerate both sodium bicarbonate and vinegar or lemon juice. This is most commonly seen in healthy children, teens, and healthy adults in their twenties, thirties, and forties (as well as a much smaller part of the adult population who are in the midlife or older age groups).

Laboratory Tests to Assess Acid-Alkaline Balance

In addition to the self-administered pH tests, there are several laboratory tests your doctor can order that will provide an indirect indication of your own acid-alkaline balance. These include hair mineral analyses and bone density studies.

Hair Mineral Analysis

Traditionally, hair mineral analysis has been used primarily to assess exposure to toxic minerals such as mercury, lead, and arsenic. For example, the technique was employed in 1961 to analyze a sample of Napoleon's hair, which was found to contain at least 100 times the usual level of arsenic considered normal, suggesting that arsenic poisoning led to his death.

Today, hair analysis is a diagnostic method used by many complementary physicians. A small sample of the newest hair growth is taken from the first inch to inch and one-half of hair starting at the scalp. This sample is then sent to a commercial lab to assess its mineral content. While mineral levels in the blood may not be representative of the amount stored in the tissues, the hair is extremely sensitive to changes in mineral reserves in the body.

Another advantage to analyzing hair rather than blood is that while the blood only contains very small amounts of minerals, making measurement more difficult, the hair contains ten to fifty times higher amounts of minerals than either blood or urine. As hair grows, minerals become part of the evolving hair protein. Several dozen trace minerals have been found in hair, including aluminum, arsenic, bromine, calcium, chlorine, cobalt, copper, iron, manganese, nickel, phosphorus, lead, sulfur, uranium, and zinc.

Bone Density Tests

Bone density scans test for osteoporosis. How porous the bones are directly reflects the decline in the reservoir of alkalinizing minerals contained within the bone to buffer excessive acids. The technology involved is similar to conventional X-rays but far more sophisticated and capable of detecting very small changes in bone density.

There are two different types of scans, single photon absorptiometry and dual-photon absorptiometry (DPA), plus an upgraded version of DPA, dual X-ray absorptiometry (DEXA). Each technique assesses different bones within the body. Single-photon absorptiometry is used to measure the density of the wrist and heel, whereas DPA and DEXA are used to assess the density of the spine and hip.

Monitoring bone density is especially important for woman as they age, as the risk of osteoporosis increases dramatically after menopause. Older men are also at greater risk of developing this condition than younger men. However, men lose bone mass much more slowly than women due to the protective benefits of testosterone.

Summary

Overacidity affects health in a wide variety of ways, from digestive problems, infectious diseases, and arthritis to such diseases as high blood pressure, osteoporosis, and cancer. Fortunately, each condition can be treated to some extent by correcting the acid-alkaline balance of the body through a combination of dietary changes and the use of alkalinizing agents.

Part 2: Restoring Your Acid-Alkaline Balance

Introduction to Part 2

This half of the book contains a very effective and powerful four-part plan that will enable you to restore your body to its healthy, slightly alkaline state. As you begin to reduce the acid load of your body and restore your mineral reserves and buffer systems and reduce the stress on your organs of elimination, you will begin to see astonishing results in your level of performance in many crucial areas. You will also begin to experience a significant improvement in your health. Your level of physical energy, mental clarity, emotional well-being, and even optimism and creativity will be enhanced as your body regains its healthful alkalinity. The frequency of respiratory illnesses like colds, flus, and sinusitis should begin to drop dramatically. Aches and pains, heartburn, allergies, and many other chronic ailments should also begin to diminish in intensity and, finally, disappear.

The four parts of this program are as follows:*

1.   Following the alkaline power diet.

2.   Restoring the alkaline mineral reserves of your cells, tissues, and bones.

3.   Using alkalinizing agents for quick symptom relief.

4.   Initiating healthy lifestyle changes to reduce the stress on your buffer systems and organs of elimination.

*Several components of this program include recommendations for nutritional supplementation. Anyone beginning a nutritional supplement program should begin at one-quarter to one-half the recommended dosages given in this book. They can then increase their dosages slowly over the course of several weeks until they have reached either the full recommended dosage or a dosage that is therapeutic for them—whichever level comes first.

Some individuals will experience therapeutic benefits at doses that are well below the doses recommended in this book.

Also, while the dosages provided in this book are appropriate for most people, there are certain groups who should continue to use less than the recommended dosages. Children, the elderly, and individuals with a frail constitution or who are extremely sensitive to drugs and nutritional supplements usually do best at therapeutic dosages of no more than half the recommended levels. Consult your physician or nutritional consultant if you have any questions about the advisability of using a particular nutritional supplement or to determine the dosage most appropriate for you.

If you follow this program carefully, symptoms of overacidity should begin to diminish quickly. Even long-standing health conditions, including chronic problems that have been present for decades, will begin to improve. If you maintain this program over time, you will rebuild your mineral reserves and restore your buffering capability. This is particularly important once you reach midlife, since most of us become progressively more acidic as part of the normal aging process. Restoring your body to its healthy, slightly alkaline pH will help you to maintain vitality and good health well into old age.

At the end of the book, I also provide a number of very important peak-performance tips for individuals who are high-alkaline producers. Unlike most of the population, these individuals actually need a diet that is both highly acidic and very nutritious. They also need acidifying nutritional supplements and medications as well as plenty of strenuous physical exercise and a fast paced, busy life to maintain a healthy pH.

6

Following the Alkaline Power Diet

The alkaline power diet will help to restore you to a naturally healthy state of slight alkalinity. By avoiding highly acidic foods and eating foods that are neutral to slightly alkaline in their pH, you will restore your reserves of alkaline minerals and other important nutrients. Equally important, this diet will decrease the wear and tear on your buffer systems and organs of elimination by reducing the acid load of the body.

This diet comprises four simple steps: (1) selecting more alkaline foods, (2) using delicious and readily available substitutions for highly acidic foods, (3) planning more alkaline meals, and (4) rotating foods for greater variety of nutrients. This diet will also cause fewer inflammatory reactions, which are extremely acidifying to the cells and tissues.

I have also included information on how to survive a binge on acidic foods, as well as guidelines on how to meet the special dietary needs of overly acidic individuals in various special groups, including athletes, corporate employees, and children and teenagers. In this section I provide much valuable information and advice that I have developed over the past two and a half decades and found to be effective for my own patients. This information will allow you to implement the alkaline power diet much more easily on your own.

Step 1: Selecting Proper Foods for the Alkaline Power Diet

First, look at the following chart showing the pH values of dozens of common foods and beverages. This chart will help you to learn the relative acidity or alkalinity of the foods that most of us eat on a daily basis. (You may be surprised at how acidic many of the foods you currently eat are.) It gives the pH of foods prior to being consumed and does not reflect the substantial acid production that some of these foods can trigger within the body. (This information is also provided in this section.) There is a lot of misinformation about the relative acidity and alkalinity of foods. Many other books have acid-alkaline food charts; however, these charts tend to contradict one another. One chart will list a food as being highly acidic, while another chart will state that the same food is highly alkaline. This can be very confusing to the reader who is trying to use this information to make intelligent choices.

My chart is based on scientific research done at major universities. This information was obtained from technical sources compiled at the University of California, Davis, Department of Food Science and Technology, and Cornell University, Department of Food Science. In addition, I obtained the pH value of certain foods from their appropriate professional associations such as the National Coffee Association. You will notice that while most food groups are listed, oils are not. Oils do not have a pH since they cannot be mixed with water, which is necessary for taking pH measurements. Many books will list pH's for oils, which is totally incorrect!

The chart will help you to plan a diet best suited to your pH needs, depending on whether you tend toward overacidity or are a naturally alkaline person. Overly acidic individuals can restore their bodies to a healthier, more alkaline state by using this chart to select foods that are less acidic and more alkaline. The chart will also indicate which foods have the highest level of acidity and should be avoided.

pH of Common Foods and Beverages
Prior to Being Consumed

Highly Acidic Foods	pH Range 1 - 4.6 Prior to Being Consumed

Beverages

Ginger ale	2.0–4.0
Lime juice	2.2–2.4
Lemon juice	2.2–2.6
Wines	2.3–3.8
Cranberry juice	2.5–2.7
Cider	2.9–3.3
Grapefruit juice	2.9–3.4
Currant juice	3.0
Orange juice	3.0–4.0
Apple juice	3.3–3.5
Pineapple juice	3.4–3.7
Prune juice	3.7–4.3
Tomato juice	3.9–4.3

Fruit

Lime	1.8–2.0
Lemon	2.2–2.4
Cranberry sauce	2.3
Gooseberries	2.8–3.1
Loquats	2.8–4.0
Orange	2.8–4.2
Plum	2.8–4.6
Rhubarb	2.9–3.4
Apple	2.9–3.5
Raspberries	2.9–3.7
Grapefruit	2.9–4.0
Boysenberries	3.0–3.3
Grapefruit sections	3.0–3.5
Strawberries	3.0–4.2
Blackberries	3.0–4.2
Kumquat	3.1–3.5
Quince	3.2
Blueberries	3.2–3.6

Highly Acidic Foods

pH Range 1 - 4.6
Prior to Being Consumed

Fruit, continued

Pineapple, crushed	3.2–4.0
Crab apples, spiced	3.3–3.7
Kiwi	3.3–3.8
Apple sauce	3.4–3.5
Apricots	3.5–4.0
Pineapple, sliced	3.5–4.1
Fruit cocktail	3.6–4.0
Raisins	3.6–4.2

Vegetables

Sauerkraut	3.1–3.7
Cucumber	3.1–3.8
Tomatillo	3.9–4.1

Dairy Products

Yogurt	3.8–4.2

Sweeteners

Fruit jellies	3.0–3.5
Fruit jams	3.5–4.0

Condiments and Seasonings

Vinegar	2.4–3.4
Pickles, sweet	2.5–3.0
Pickles, dill	2.6–3.8
Pickles, sour	3.0–3.5
Fermented olives	3.5
Mayonnaise	3.8–4.0

Moderately Acidic Foods

pH Range 3.1 – 5.6 Prior to Being Consumed

Beverages

Beer	4.0–5.0

Fruit

Peach	3.1–4.7
Cherries	3.2–4.7
Pear	3.4–4.7
Mango	3.9–4.6
Asian pear	4.2–4.6
Guava	4.3–4.7
Banana	4.5–5.2

Vegetables

Tomato	3.7–4.9
Potato salad	3.9–4.6
Eggplant	4.5–4.7
String beans	4.6

Red Meat

Dry sausage	4.4–5.6

Dairy Products

Cottage cheese	4.1–5.4

Condiments and Seasonings

Fermented vegetables	3.9–5.1
Red pimento	4.3–5.2

Low Acid to Alkaline Foods	pH Range 4.6 – 9.5 Prior to Being Consumed
Beverages	
Coffee	4.9–5.2
Mineral water	6.2–9.4
Distilled water	6.8–7.0
Fruit	
Figs	4.6–5.0
Papaya	5.2–5.7
Persimmon	5.4–5.8
Avocado	5.5–6.0
Dates	6.2–6.4
Cantaloupe	6.2–6.5
Melon	6.3–6.7
Vegetables	
Pumpkin	4.8–5.5
Sweet pepper	4.8–6.0
Spinach	4.8–6.8
Carrot	4.9–6.3
Squash	5.0–5.4

Asparagus	5.0–6.1
Turnip	5.2–5.6
Cabbage	5.2–6.3
Broccoli	5.2–6.5
Parsnip	5.3
Sweet potato	5.3–5.6
Onion	5.3–5.8
Peas	5.3–6.8
Turnip greens	5.4–5.6
White potato	5.4–6.3
Artichoke	5.6
Cauliflower	5.6–6.7
Parsley	5.7–6.0
Celery	5.7–6.1
Alfalfa tops	5.9
Corn	5.9–7.3
Lettuce	6.0–6.4
Mushrooms	6.0–6.5
Brussels sprout	6.3–6.6

Low Acid to Alkaline Foods	pH Range 4.6 – 9.5 Prior to Being Consumed

Beans

Baked beans	4.8–5.5
Dried beans	4.9–5.5
Kidney	5.2–5.4
Lima	5.4–6.5
Soybeans	6.0–6.6

Nuts and Seeds

Walnuts	5.4–5.5
Almonds	> 6.0
Flax seeds	> 6.0
Hazelnuts	> 6.0
Pecans	> 6.0
Poppy seeds	> 6.0
Pumpkin seeds	> 6.0
Sesame seeds	> 6.0
Sunflower seeds	> 6.0

Fish and Shellfish

Halibut	5.5–5.8
Sardines	5.7–6.6
Tuna	5.9–6.1
Mackerel	5.9–6.2
Oysters	5.9–6.7
Clams	5.9–7.1
Codfish (canned)	6.0–6.1
Salmon	6.1–6.5
Haddock	6.2–6.7
Whiting	6.2–7.1
Catfish	6.6–7.0
Scallops	6.8–7.1
Crab	6.8–8.0
Shrimp	6.8–8.2

Low Acid to Alkaline Foods

**pH Range 4.6 – 9.5
Prior to Being Consumed**

Poultry

Chicken	5.5–6.4
Duck	6.0–6.1
Egg yolk	6.0–6.3
Egg white	7.9–9.5

Red Meat

Beef	5.3–6.2
Pork	5.3–6.4
Corned-beef hash	5.5–6.0
Spiced ham	6.0–6.3
Hot dogs	6.2

Dairy Products

Roquefort cheese	4.7–4.8
Most cheeses	5.0–6.1
Parmesan cheese	5.2–5.3
Evaporated milk	5.9–6.3
Whole cow's milk	6.0–6.8
Butter	6.1–6.4

Grains

Wheat	> 6.0
Rice	> 6.0
Barley	> 6.0
Oats	> 6.0
Rye	> 6.0
Millet	> 6.0
Quinoa	> 6.0
Amaranth	> 6.0
Hominy	6.9–7.9

Baked Goods

White bread	5.0–6.0
Date-nut bread	5.1–6.0
Soda crackers	6.5–8.5

Sweeteners

Molasses	5.0–5.4
Glucose syrup	5.2
Honey	6.0–6.8
Brown-rice syrup	6.1–6.4
Maple syrup	6.5–7.0

Condiments and Seasonings

Hot peppers	4.8–6.0
Garlic	5.3–6.3
Cocoa	5.5–6.0
Ripe, canned olives	5.9–7.3
Dutch processed chocolate	7.0–8.0

Eat a More Alkaline Diet

If you have symptoms of overacidity, it is important to eat foods listed in the "Low Acid to Alkaline" section of the chart. Eating foods such as vegetables, grains, beans, small amounts of raw seeds and nuts, and fish and shellfish will help to lessen the acid load of the body and reduce the wear and tear on the pH-regulating systems as well as the organs of elimination. Ground, raw flax meal deserves a special mention as a rich source of both alkaline minerals and anti-inflammatory omega-3 oils. Flax meal can be used in blender drinks and as a cereal.

If you are overly acidic, eating these foods will begin to enhance your performance in many areas of your life as well as increase your physical energy, stamina, and resistance to disease. The more alkaline foods are higher in nutrients and are full of the alkaline minerals needed to restore the alkaline reserves in your cells, tissues, and bones. These foods also tend to be less allergenic and less likely to cause inflammatory reactions, which acidify your cells.

The alkaline power diet has enormous variety and includes a tremendous range of flavors. Its major food groups include vegetables, starches, gluten-free grains, legumes (beans and peas), seeds, nuts, fish, sea vegetables, and fruits like papaya and melons. Besides helping to restore your performance capability, the alkaline power diet provides many health benefits such as reducing the risk of heart attacks and strokes, cancer, and crippling, inflammatory conditions like arthritis.

Your diet and food selection should concentrate on foods that have a pH above 5.0. This will create a diet that has a vegetarian emphasis but includes rich sources of proteins like legumes, whole grains, raw seeds and nuts, and fish and shellfish. Fish and shellfish do not have the tough, fibrous protein found in red meat. As a result, the stomach produces less hydrochloric acid to digest these foods than is necessary for the breakdown of red meat.

Fish such as salmon, mackerel, trout, and tuna also contain anti-inflammatory polyunsaturated oils rather than the inflammatory saturated fats found in red meat and dairy products. Because of the accumulation of mercury, they should not be eaten more than twice a week. In addition, mercury free fish or algae based omega-3 oils can be taken as a supplement for daily use.

Most people eat seeds and nuts salted, fried in oil, or coated with sugar. These are popular snack foods while watching TV or movies, sitting in airplanes, or socializing in cocktail lounges. Instead of partaking of these snacks, bring your own raw organic seeds and nuts as highly nutritious, low-acid alternatives.

Avoid Highly Acidic Foods and Acid-Forming Foods

More than 90 percent of Americans become overly acidic during their lifetime due, in part, to the foods they eat. The amount of overly acidic foods consumed each day in the United States is staggering, especially when you consider that a person needs a slightly alkaline pH to be able to perform to their best and remain in optimal health. The damage that these highly acidic foods inflict on the body was traditionally demonstrated in high-school experiments in which a tooth is placed in a glass of cola and allowed to remain there for several weeks or months. Within a relatively short period of time, the tooth begins to dissolve.

When taken into our bodies, these same cola drinks would inflict similar damage if they were not neutralized by our pH-regulating systems. While colas are a synthetic creation, there are many extremely popular natural foods that we eat that have pHs that are similar to or even lower than cola drinks, including limes, lemons, orange juice, most berries, cranberry sauce, vinegar, dill and sweet pickles, jams and jellies, and wine.

If you have an overly acidic constitution, the constant consumption of highly acidic food will, over time, rob you of your energy and vitality, reduce your mental clarity, and even dampen your optimism and enthusiasm for life. You may experience a slowdown in your ability to recover from injuries, surgery, and strenuous physical activities.

The overconsumption of acidic foods can also cause you to become more prone to infections, runny noses, and allergic reactions. You may also notice an increase in aches and pains. I have had many overly acidic patients tell her that drinking a glass of orange juice triggered heartburn, drinking a cup of coffee caused bladder discomfort, and eating dairy products triggered nasal congestion.

As you look at the chart showing the pH values of common foods and beverages, you will probably be surprised at how many commonly eaten foods are highly acidic. Examples of the various acids contained within our daily fare include acetic acid, which gives vinegar its tartness, and citric acid, found in oranges, lemons, and limes. Carbonated soft drinks bubble because they are infused with carbon dioxide, a highly acidic substance that is actually a waste product of our own metabolism. A major component of tea is tannic acid.

Caffeinated coffee contains many volatile acids, which are particularly abundant in gourmet blends and provide coffee with its desirable rich flavor. Red meat, dairy products, and soft drinks are high in acidic minerals like sulfur and phosphorus (which are converted to sulfuric acid and phosphoric acid).

Many of these foods are not necessarily "bad." For example, citrus fruits contain vitamin C in the juice and bioflavonoids, which are beneficial antioxidants, in the pulp. They also contain small amounts of alkaline minerals such as potassium (unlike the juices of the other, more tart citrus fruits like lemon, orange and tangerine juices are actually rich sources of the alkaline mineral potassium, despite their low pH).

In fact, in traditional folk medicine there is a myth that, lemon juice and vinegar (particularly cider vinegar) are frequently recommended to detoxify the body and as alkalinizing agents, in part because of their purported alkalinity. However, the actual alkaline mineral content of lemon juice and cider vinegar is very low and does not counter their intrinsic acid content.

In addition, the low pH of these two delicious and useful condiments indicates that they are actually highly acidic and, like all acidic foods, must be buffered when eaten to neutralize their low pH and to bring them up to the slightly alkaline pH of the body. Like all acidic foods, foods like lemon juice and apple cider vinegar do become alkaline when eaten. But this is at the expense of our body's buffering system.

Each of the trillions of cells in your body contain many alkaline substances—minerals such as calcium, magnesium, potassium, and sodium, as well as oxygen and bicarbonate. The combination of all these substances produces a slightly alkaline pH within your cells. Your body's internal functions—including energy production, immunity, and much of your digestive process—work most efficiently in this alkaline environment.

In addition to your cells, your blood must also maintain a slightly alkaline state in order for your body to function efficiently. Unfortunately, you—and your blood and cells—are constantly exposed to a variety of acidic substances, including environmental pollutants, acidic or acid-forming foods like lemon juice and apple cider vinegar, and even stress. To help neutralize the acidity caused by these daily offenders, your body has a complex buffering system that works hard to maintain alkalinity.

However, as most people age, this buffering system weakens, causing excess acid to be neutralized less effectively. This contributes to decreased energy levels, reduced immunity, and increased risk of diseases, such as osteoporosis. Since your bones contain high amounts of alkaline minerals, like calcium and magnesium, your body draws these substances from your bones to help alkalinize the rest of your system. Over time, this leaching of minerals can lead to bone loss.

As a result, lemon juice and cider vinegar are best used as detoxification or purification remedies only by high-alkaline producers or individuals with healthy buffering capabilities (usually younger adults in their twenties, thirties, and forties), for whom frequent doses or large quantities may be prescribed and well tolerated. If you need to increase your intake of alkaline minerals, you are better off using more-alkaline, high-pH condiments or even multimineral supplements. The accompanying chart compares the pH and mineral content of lemon juice and cider vinegar with other, more-alkaline condiments and flavoring agents.

pH and Alkaline Mineral Content of Common Flavoring Agents and Condiments (per tablespoon)

Food	pH	Calcium	Magnesium	Potassium	Sodium
Lemon juice	2.2–2.6	2 mg	1 mg	15 mg	3 mg
Lime juice	2.2–2.4	1 mg	1 mg	17 mg	0 mg
Cider vinegar	2.4–3.4	0.8 mg	3 mg	14 mg	trace
Blackstrap Molasses	5.0–5.4	137 mg	52 mg	585 mg	19 mg
Tahini (sesame paste)	> 6.0	64 mg	14 mg	110 mg	17 mg
Flax meal	> 6.0	35 mg	63 mg	120 mg	7 mg
Kelp	(n/a)	156 mg	104 mg	4.5 mg	11.5 mg

In my clinical practice, I have found that the ingestion of more-acidic, low-pH foods such as citrus fruits and juices and different types of vinegars can be incredibly stressful to overly acidic persons despite these foods' potential nutritional benefits. The reason for this is that their highly acidic pH can trigger either immediate or slower-acting stress responses within the body.

For example, many of my overly acidic patients have frequently complained about citrus fruits and vinegar causing unpleasant reactions like canker sores, heartburn and joint discomfort. Other potentially nutritious but highly acidic foods like tomatoes, pineapple and wine can also cause similar symptoms. Repeated consumption of these low-pH foods tends to trigger chronic damage, inflammation and overacidity in affected tissues of sensitive people.

Interestingly, these symptoms can occur in some individuals even before the food has left the stomach. This suggests that a nonchemical process may be taking place since the pH-regulating systems of the body cannot work this rapidly. To explain this phenomenon, some researchers have suggested that certain stress factors, like the overacidity of foods, may cause an immediate electrical imbalance within the body, which is then followed by the actual chemical responses to the stressor agent.

In contrast, high-alkaline producers or younger individuals with healthy and intact buffering capability may actually benefit from the wide variety of beneficial nutrients contained within highly acidic foods. Such individuals can handle these foods' low pH without their causing negative side effects. For example, certain fruit juices that are high in potassium citrate and alkaline salts of citric acid can be used to maintain energy and stamina while participating in athletic activities. Such drinks are best used by high-alkaline producers who can tolerate their high content of simple sugar and do not develop tissue reactions such as canker sores, heartburn, and other types of irritation from the use of these drinks.

Whether acid or alkaline in their pH prior to ingestion, many foods can also generate a tremendous amount of acid within the body once they are eaten. For example, protein-rich foods of animal origin, like red meat and dairy products, or tough plant protein like the gluten contained in wheat, rye, barley, and oats can stimulate the stomach to produce large amounts of hydrochloric acid, which is needed to begin the breakdown of these proteins. In addition, coffee, alcohol, and fast foods like pizza can also trigger significant hydrochloric-acid production.

Many foods also cause overacidity, because they trigger either food allergies or specific sensitivities in susceptible individuals (see the following chart). Milk products, wheat, soy, peanuts, and eggs are examples of common foods that contain proteins to which the body can mount an exaggerated immune response in susceptible people. Many individuals are also allergic to sulfites (see the following chart). These are chemicals used as preservatives in canned, frozen, and otherwise processed foods. Other foods like tomatoes, oranges, wine, and chocolate as well as the sugars found in milk (lactose) or fruits (fructose) can trigger symptoms of overacidity in individuals who have sensitivities to these foods or lack the enzymes needed to digest them.

Finally, many foods—such as red meat (including hamburgers and hot dogs), dairy products, margarine, coconut oil, and palm kernel oil—contain saturated fats, which can cause highly acidic, inflammatory reactions within the body. Foods that trigger allergies, sensitivities, or inflammation within the body can damage tissue far from the site of ingestion. The joints, skin, bladder, reproductive organs, and thyroid are but a few of the organs and tissues that can incur injury due to improper food selection. Over time, chronic damage to and injury of the affected cells and tissues can lead to reduced energy production, a decrease in oxygen levels, and a loss of alkaline substances and minerals—all of which can contribute to overacidity and, ultimately, disease.

Foods That Commonly Cause Allergies

Dairy products
Wheat
Citrus fruits
Strawberries
Rye
Pork
Corn

Nuts
Soybeans
Shellfish
Chocolate
Eggs
Tomatoes

Foods That Tend to Contain Sulfites*

Potato chips	Scallops
Carrots	Coleslaw
Soups (canned or dry)	Shrimp
Tomatoes	Beer
Mushrooms (canned or fresh)	Oysters
Peppers	Wine
Pickles	Clams
Potatoes	Cider
French fries (frozen)	Lobster
	Lettuce

*Sulfites are used as preservatives and sanitizing agents in food processing. Many individuals have adverse reactions to sulfites.

If liver function is impaired and the liver is unable to fully detoxify certain components of our diet, acidic by-products will accumulate. Alcohol, red meat, dairy products, pizza, peanuts, and cashews, among other foods, are hard for the liver to process. Finally, most foods are broken down into acidic waste products, which must be neutralized and then eliminated from the body. Not surprisingly, all of these by-products and waste products can greatly add to the acid load of the body and produce a constant and ongoing stress on our buffer systems and organs of elimination. As a result, everyone except high-alkaline producers has the deck stacked against them when eating the standard American diet.

How to Modify Common Acidic Foods and Dishes

I have included the following tips to enable you to still enjoy some of the highly acidic but nutritious foods that you may currently be eating. While high-alkaline producers can eat these foods as a regular part of their diet, overly acidic individuals cannot.

Fruit drinks. Many overly acidic people would like to enjoy blenderized fruit drinks and smoothies because of their delicious taste and high nutrient content. Unfortunately, the high level of acidity of many fruits can cause canker sores, heartburn, abdominal discomfort, and even a drop in energy in overly acidic people.

To neutralize the acidity of the fruit, I recommend using a product called Acid Check, which is gradually released into your body. It is a mixture containing potassium, magnesium, and calcium that comes in granular and caplet form. I recommend 2 to 3 caplets per day or if you prefer granules mix 1/4 teaspoon into 4-8 ounces of water two times a day between meals.

The granular form comes in a shaker bottle, so you can also use it on the spot to neutralize highly acidic foods such as tomatoes, citrus fruits and juices, berries, salad dressings, spicy foods, sugary foods, and wine. The granules do not alter the flavor or aroma of foods or beverages it's sprinkled but it may make them taste sweeter due to the reduced acid content. Consider keeping a bottle with you for restaurant meals, special occasions, and other times when you don't have as much control over what you eat and need to reduce the meal acidity by as much as 90%.

I also recommend using 2 to 3 caplets per day to promote healthy alkalinization or, if you prefer the granules, mix 1/4 teaspoon into 4-8 ounces of water two times a day between meals. You can purchase Acid Check at www.acidcheck.com.

For best digestibility, these drinks should be consumed by themselves on an empty stomach, preferably in the morning. If you wish to add protein powder to this drink, use vegetable protein derived from rice or legumes, which are less acidic than animal protein. In addition, do not consume this drink with a protein-rich meal containing meat or milk, since these proteins require more acid production within the stomach for their digestion.

Wine. Many overly acidic individuals would love to drink an occasional glass of wine but find that it causes heartburn and other digestive symptoms. This is because wine has an acidic pH. The alcohol contained within wine also triggers the production of hydrochloric acid within the stomach. As with the fruit drinks, you can use Acid Check granules to bring up the pH of the wine and neutralize its acidity.

For special social occasions, you can take sodium bicarbonate (baking soda) or a sodium and potassium bicarbonate mixture right after drinking an alcoholic beverage to blunt its acidic effect on the body. Bicarbonate can also be used to help neutralize the uncomfortable symptoms of an alcohol-induced hangover.

Coffee and tea. If you feel you cannot live without your daily cup of coffee or black tea, add Acid Check to your favorite cup of coffee or black tea.

Sparkling water. If you are at a bar or restaurant and want to drink mineral water but only bubbling varieties are available, you can get rid of the carbonation by adding a pinch of table salt. This will allow the water to go flat, leaving you with a more alkaline drink.

Salad dressings. You can substitute Bragg Liquid Aminos for vinegar when making salad dressings. Bragg Liquid Aminos is a delicious flavoring agent that can be purchased in most health food stores. Combine it with olive oil and herbs for a delicious dressing. Alternatively, you can prepare a salad dressing by decreasing the amount of vinegar by half and increasing the amount of water and oil, as well as by adding extra flavoring agents such as herbs.

Marinated vegetables. Avoid vegetables marinated in vinegar. These are highly acidic and are commonly served in Italian and Spanish restaurants and occasionally in American ones. Many restaurants offer alternative vegetable appetizers such as steamed artichokes or asparagus. You can also order small side dishes of whatever cooked vegetables are being served that day.

Salt. Sea vegetables are rich in minerals and can be used to replace the more acidic table salt as a flavoring agent. Sea vegetables are now available in shakers to be used as a condiment in natural-food stores.

Step 2: Making Substitutions in Your Diet

Once you know which foods are either high in acid or become so after being eaten, and which foods are more alkaline, you can begin to substitute the more alkaline foods for the ones that are causing you to become acidic.

Replace Acid Foods with Less Acidic/More Alkaline Ones

One of the most difficult obstacles we all face when making dietary changes is the prospect of giving up foods we really love. In fact, the inability to give up things we find enjoyable is often the biggest barrier to making changes that can lead to long-term improvements in health and performance. Now that you have had a chance to review the pH values of many common foods, you may find that some of your most enjoyable and "can't live without" foods are in the highly acidic category.

These are foods that either contain high levels of acid before we ingest them, like lemon juice and vinegar, or cause acid to be produced in the body after we eat them, like red meat, dairy products, and wheat. Many of these are probably foods that you have eaten all your life, and you may be reluctant to give them up because you enjoy their flavor, taste, or texture.

Fortunately, you can replace a highly acidic food or beverage with a similar one that is more alkaline. The trick is to do this with a substitution that retains a similarly pleasurable flavor yet is also high in nutrients. For example, you can use soy- or rice-based frozen desserts instead of ice cream, or vegetarian patties instead of hamburgers. To help familiarize you with the substitution options that are available, I have developed the following chart which lists many highly acidic foods as well as their less acidic, more alkaline substitutes.

In recent years there have been incredible improvements in the quality, taste, and appearance of food substitutes. This has primarily occurred as the demand for low-fat food substitutes has increased. More recently, foods have been developed to meet the demand for alternatives to foods that are known to be highly allergenic, such as wheat and dairy products.

While none of these substitutes was originally developed to restore pH balance, you can use many of them for this purpose because they also happen to be much less acidic than the foods they replace (soy is a notable exception: many individuals are soy intolerant and should avoid soy-containing foods). The market for these substitutes is growing rapidly, with many companies now competing for shelf space. Therefore, the quality is continuing to improve as food technologists are continually making refinements in taste and texture.

Initially, these products were of very poor quality, with the carton often tasting better than the product inside. Today, however, there are substitutes for cheese that both taste and melt the way real cheese does. There are substitutes for wheat pasta (such as rice, corn, and quinoa) that taste like the pasta you grew up with. There are also substitutes for meat and dairy products that are hard to tell from the originals. In fact, I have made nachos for my daughter and her friends with nondairy cheese that are so tasty that they had no idea they weren't eating real cheese. If these foods can pass the "kid test," then you can feel comfortable giving them a try.

These substitutes are now easy to find in health food stores, many supermarkets, and a surprising number of restaurants. Garden burgers are now being served in many restaurants, and you can order pizzas made with vegetarian-based soy and rice cheeses. Given the improvement in flavor and texture, any overly acidic person can enjoy these substitutes whether they are cooking for themselves, dining out, or preparing meals for an entire family. I have been recommending these food substitutes to my patients for years and have seen excellent results. With the many different brands available, you should be able to find substitutes that appeal to your taste.

Use Substitutes in Cooking

You can reinvent an old-favorite recipe with new, more alkalinizing ingredients. Check the following chart and see where you can make some of these substitutions and have a favorite recipe become a much less acidic dish. You can also start with one of the appetizing new food products, such as mozzarella-like cheese substitutes made with soy, and create a homemade pizza that is far more alkalinizing and healthful than the dairy-based version. Pancakes, cheesecake, and fettuccine Alfredo can also be made with substitute ingredients and are quite delicious and more healthful since they are not as acid forming within the body. Review the chart and purchase one of the substitutes each time you shop. Try them in your favorite recipes, and you will soon have a number of less acidic food substitutes to choose from.

Make Substitutions at Your Own Speed

As with any habit or pattern, one's personal preference for how best to initiate a change will vary from person to person. Some people prefer to make changes all at once and will immediately adopt a completely nonmeat, nondairy, vegetarian diet. Others prefer to ease themselves slowly into dietary changes and will begin to add new foods and substitutions gradually, while reducing the frequency and portion size of many of their favorite and highly acidic foods. Choose the method that suits you best.

Even after a healthier, more alkaline pH has been restored to the cells and tissues, a person who tends to have an acidic constitution will probably have to continue a more alkaline diet for the rest of their lives. However, as with most things, you will become accustomed to the new way of eating, enjoying the many benefits of increased energy and stamina. Before long, highly acidic foods such as greasy French fries or pizza with extra cheese and meat toppings will no longer seem as appealing.

A Warning on Substituting Foods

If you know you are allergic or find that you are sensitive to any of the food substitutes listed, do not use them as they will cause an acidic inflammatory reaction in your body and defeat their purpose. This situation is seen most often in individuals who are allergic to soy products, as mentioned above.

Alkalinizing Food Supplements

Spirulina and other green foods are nutrient rich and promote alkalinity within the body. They are an excellent source of many easily absorbable, alkaline minerals as well as amino acids, vitamins, enzymes, and chlorophyll, and can be used to supplement your regular meals. The following is a list of green foods commonly found on the market:

Spirulina and chlorella are microalgae that provide a concentrated source of protein containing all the amino acids and are a good source of minerals as well.

Green magma, made from young barley leaves, supplies amino acids and minerals.

Kyo-green, a combination of barley, wheatgrass, kelp, and chlorella, provides amino acids and many nutrients.

Alfalfa is a source of abundant calcium, magnesium, phosphorus, and potassium in a balanced ratio that promotes absorption.

Barley grass is an excellent source of all the amino acids, calcium, and iron.

Food Substitutes for Highly Acidic or Acid-Forming Foods

Natural-food stores carry many of the following substitute foods, and even supermarkets carry some of these products.

Highly Acidic Foods	Less Acidic, Alkaline Food Substitutes
Wheat Products	
Wheat bread	Bread made with brown rice, millet, amaranth, quinoa, soy*, oat and nut flours
Wheat crackers	Brown rice, corn, potato and nut based crackers
Wheat pasta	Brown rice, corn, quinoa and buckwheat pasta
Wheat waffles	Brown rice waffles
Wheat cookies	Brown nice, quinoa, and millet and nut flour cookies
Dairy Products	
Cow's milk	Soy*, rice, multigrain, nut, coconut, flax and hemp milks
Cheese	Soy*, rice and almond cheeses
Ice cream	Frozen desserts made with rice, coconut, almond or soy* milk
Yogurt	Soy*, almond, or coconut yogurt

Highly Acidic Foods	Less Acidic, Alkaline Food Substitutes
Meat Products	
Beef, pork, and lamb	Fish, shellfish, and free-range poultry, vegetarian meat substitutes and occasional free-range red meat and game
Hamburger	Chicken, turkey, tofu, soy* and garden burgers
Hot dogs, sausage	Chicken, turkey, tofu, soy*and garden burgers
Meat loaf	Multigrain and legume loaves
Fried and Fatty Foods	
Deep-fried corn chips	Baked corn chips, rice, potato and nut chips
Pizza made with a wheat crust	Pizza made with a brown rice flour crust and nondairy cheese
Sweeteners	
Refined white sugar	Xylitol, agave syrup, maple syrup, coconut palm sugar, brown-rice syrup, honey

Beverages

Coffee	Grain-based coffee substitutes
Black tea, green tea	Herbal teas such as peppermint, chamomile and rose hips
Soft drinks and fruit juices	Mineral water

Condiments and Flavorings

Vinegar	Bragg Liquid Aminos**
Mayonnaise	Safflower oil, tofu–based mayonnaise
Ketchup	Sugar-free ketchup
Salt	Garlic, fresh herbs, sea vegetables, lemon rind, Bragg Liquid Aminos**

*Soy products such as tofu, soymilk, and soy flour can be acid-forming for individuals with soy allergy.

**Bragg Liquid Aminos is a seasoning agent available in health food stores.

Step 3: Meal Planning

While you are following a program to restore your body to a more alkaline pH, proper food selection is critical to avoid putting undue wear and tear on your already stressed buffer systems. See the chart below for sample menus that you can use as a model for meal planning at home.

Typical Alkalinizing Meals

Breakfast

Puffed-rice cereal
Rice, soy or other nondairy milk
Papaya slices
Peppermint tea

Pancakes made with non-gluten flour mix such as rice, tapioca or soy flour, topped with flax seed oil, small amount of substitute sweetener
Melon
Grain-based coffee substitute

Garden vegetable omelette
Rice toast with flax seed oil
Vegetable juice

Tofu scramble with onions, mushrooms and green peppers
Millet or rice toast with nondairy butter
Chamomile Tea

Nondairy yogurt

Blueberries and strawberries

Rice cake with almond butter

Lunch

Lentil soup

Grilled vegan cheddar cheese sandwich on rice bread

Coleslaw with cabbage, carrots and beets

Mineral water

Garden burger, lettuce, tomato and onion

Mixed greens salad

Baked sweet potato fries

Mineral water

Chef's salad with mixed greens, tuna, kidney beans, hard-boiled egg

Quinoa muffin

Rose hip tea

Split-pea soup

Rice pasta

Baked yam and steamed kale

Blueberry tea

Dinner

Vegetable and navy bean soup

Mixed field greens salad with vinaigrette dressing

Rice crackers

Mineral water

Tostada with a corn tortilla, kidney beans, rice, avocado, grilled onion and cilantro

Ginger tea

Rice tabbouleh

Hummus

Romaine lettuce salad with herb vinaigrette dressing

Mineral water with lemon

Broiled tuna

Quinoa with mixed vegetables

Steamed broccoli with Bragg Liquid Aminos* and flaxseed oil

Peppermint tea

Broiled salmon

Baked potato

Steamed kale with Bragg Liquid Aminos* and olive oil

Chamomile tea

*Bragg Liquid Aminos is a seasoning agent available in health food stores.

Choosing Less Acidic/More Alkaline Meals in Restaurants

Traditionally, people have chosen mostly highly acidic dishes and entrées when eating in restaurants. Luckily, all-American fare such as the 16 oz. porterhouse steak, French fries, and rich, sugary deserts, and French cuisine with its heavy butter- and cream-based sauces have been replaced or supplemented in many restaurants by lighter, healthier, and less acidic, more alkaline dishes. This is true both in American restaurants and in those serving ethnic cuisines. The important thing is to know which dishes on the menu represent the less acidic, more alkaline options and to select a variety of such dishes when dining out.

I have prepared the following list to assist you in making intelligent menu selections, particularly if you are working hard to restore your body to a healthier, more alkaline state. In general, you will want to order salads, nondairy soups, vegetable or bean appetizers and side dishes, and vegetarian or fish entrées. Remember, most restaurants are willing to make up vegetarian entrées and platters at your request, even if they are not on the menu.

American cuisine: salad or salad bars, bean or vegetable soups, baked potatoes, rice, vegetable side dishes or platters, fish or shellfish entrées.

Italian cuisine: escarole soup, bean or minestrone soup, white bean salad, Caesar salad, risotto, polenta (cornmeal) with a mushroom sauce, grilled eggplant entrée, fish or shellfish entrées.

French cuisine: vegetable or seafood salads, nondairy soups, vegetable side dishes, stewed beans, fish or shellfish entrées.

Indian cuisine: lentils, rice pilafs, cucumber salad, curried vegetable or shellfish dishes.

Chinese cuisine: stir-fried vegetables, sizzling rice soup, tofu or bean curd dishes, steamed rice, shrimp and mixed vegetable entrées.

Japanese cuisine: Japanese salads, miso soup, sticky rice, sushi, side dishes and soups made with vegetables and tofu.

Mexican cuisine: mixed vegetable salads, tostada salad, bean and rice side dishes, bean or shrimp burritos, bean or seafood tacos.

How Overly Acidic and Naturally Alkaline People Can Dine Well Together

Married couples and members of the same family can have different acid-alkaline constitutions and may require different food choices. One spouse may be overly acidic while the other is a high-alkaline producer. Children's acid-alkaline balance may differ from that of their parents. This same issue can also arise when socializing with friends or business associates. Since the standard American diet is so prevalent, overly acidic people will often try to keep up with their more alkaline spouse or friend, much to their detriment. It is important to eat according to the needs of your basic constitution: You will feel better and maintain your health more readily if you stick to the diet best suited to your pH needs.

This is not as difficult as you might expect. When cooking at home, overly acidic and more alkaline individuals can share soups, salads, vegetable dishes, and starches. Their entrées, however, may differ. A more alkaline individual may choose to eat meat as an entrée much more frequently and often in larger portions. Remember, high-alkaline producers need to do this to maintain their level of energy. Overly acidic people should choose grain- and legume-based entrées instead with occasional servings of fish and poultry eaten in smaller amounts.

My overly acidic patients have reported that customizing entrées while keeping all of the side dishes the same is really not too difficult. Sometimes, they will even prepare food for the whole family—like spaghetti and meatballs, tacos, and casseroles—and simply not add the red meat to their portions.

In addition, overly acidic people may want to skip the vinegar marinades and dressings, wheat bread, wine, coffee, and dessert that their naturally alkaline dining partner(s) can enjoy in moderation. Luckily, these individuals can enjoy the many substitutions that are now available and not feel deprived. For example, slices of very tasty rice bread can be served alongside the wheat bread. Or garden burgers can be prepared on the grill right next to the all-beef hamburgers.

Restaurant dining is somewhat easier when people with different acid-alkaline constitutions eat together, because a restaurant menu normally contains many more dishes than are prepared for one meal at home. On the negative side, diners have no control over the ingredients used to prepare a dish or the types of dishes offered.

While your naturally alkaline dining partner may choose to order a highly vinegary antipasti followed by steak with a glass of red wine and an apple tart for dessert, an overly acidic person can put together a tasty and varied meal by ordering a vegetable soup, salad, and several vegetable side dishes or rice-based dishes or fish as an entrée. This allows for great flexibility in both ordering and eating. And if you and your dining partner are willing to share your dishes, all the better. When you order a broccoli and beef dish in a Chinese restaurant, for example, the acidic diner can eat most of the broccoli while the alkaline one eats most of the beef.

Step 4: Rotate Your Foods

Food allergies and food sensitivities are frequently seen in many overly acidic individuals. Food allergies occur when an individual has an exaggerated immune-system response to specific proteins found in various foods. The body's immune system reacts to these foods as if they were foreign invaders, much like the viruses and bacteria that can cause disease.

The allergic reaction will trigger an outpouring of inflammatory substances that cause cells and tissues to become overly acidic. This can cause a runny nose, itching and tearing of the eyes, swelling of the sinuses, tightness in the throat, coughing, wheezing, skin rashes, fatigue, anxiety, and a host of other symptoms. Approximately 25 percent of the population is estimated to have wheat and dairy allergies. Millions of other individuals have specific intolerances to these same foods, due to enzyme deficiencies and the inability to properly digest them.

Other foods such as peanuts, corn, soy, eggs, and chocolate can also trigger an allergic reaction in sensitive individuals. In addition, the milk or nuts used in preparing chocolate products can also cause the sensitivity reaction. While fish and shellfish are highly recommended as primary sources of protein in the alkaline power diet, they should be avoided in individuals with sensitivities to these foods. When an allergic reaction to any food occurs, the cells become more acidic.

Many other foods also cause overacidity in the body because individuals lack the enzymes needed to digest them. The best example of this is lactose intolerance. Lactose is a sugar found in milk that cannot be digested by 70 to 100 percent of blacks, Asians, and Native Americans and 60 to 90 percent of Mediterranean populations. Many individuals are also sensitive to fructose, or fruit sugar, which is found in thousands of food products. Finally, foods that contain amines (monosodium glutamate, or MSG, being the best known) are also irritating to the body. Amines are found in tomatoes, bananas, oranges, wine, chocolate, mushrooms, and Parmesan cheese.

Unfortunately, most overly acidic individuals tend to crave the foods that they are allergic to or have specific intolerances for. They will often eat these foods on a repetitive basis, sometimes consuming them every day for months or even years. This type of eating stresses the immune system and constantly triggers an allergic or sensitivity reaction within the body, leading to symptoms that are both uncomfortable and chronic.

To break this pattern and reduce the amount of overacidity being constantly created within the body, try rotating your foods so that they are eaten, at most, once every four days. A four-day rotational diet will greatly reduce your sensitivity to foods that you may be allergic to, thereby reducing acidic, inflammatory reactions within the body. For example, a typical rotation might alternate beans, fish, and eggs, with grain- and vegetable-based burgers, casseroles, and loaves as primary sources of protein.

All foods should be rotated on this program, including your beverages, condiments, and oils. People who eat a rotational diet tend to eat fresh, unprocessed foods, which change seasonally as different crops are planted and harvested. This type of eating provides a much greater variety of alkaline nutrients and essential nutrients than eating the same thing every day. Some individuals choose to eat the same foods day after day simply because they do not like to cook or feel that they do not have time to prepare food due to a very busy work and social schedule.

Fortunately, health food stores, delis, and supermarkets often serve less acidic food options like falafel, hummus, Garden burgers, roasted chicken, broiled salmon, grilled shrimp, and a wide variety of salads and even vegan mashed potatoes, grilled vegetables, and vegetable purees, all of which can be taken home and eaten. Garden burgers can be cooked in a skillet or oven at home and are ready to eat in a few minutes. Be sure the inside temperature has reached at least 165 degrees. Similarly, fish can be simply broiled or grilled with no more preparation involved than sprinkling on a few herbs.

Surviving an Occasional Binge of Highly Acidic Foods

All of us are occasionally invited to birthday parties, weddings, bar mitzvahs, Christmas parties, and Thanksgiving dinners, where virtually every food served is highly acidic and tempting to the eye and taste buds. Such festivities and holiday celebrations tend to include champagne, canapés, roast beef, ham, and beautifully prepared desserts. On these occasions, even the most overly acidic person will want to throw caution to the wind and eat, drink, and be merry. However, no one likes to wake up the next morning with an acid stomach, hangover, brain fog, or even a runny nose and aching joints from seriously overindulging on these highly acidic foods.

To minimize the deleterious effects that an occasional binge on highly acidic foods can cause, you can pursue the following program before, during, and after the binge itself. A half hour before you plan to eat, take the following nutritional supplements: 1 to 3 g of buffered vitamin C, one to two pancreatic digestive enzyme tablets, 500 mg of bromelain, a plant-based digestive enzyme, and 50 to 100 mg of vitamin B complex. With the meal, take one or two more pancreatic enzymes tablets and an additional bromelain tablet.

One hour to one and one-half hour after eating, take one-half teaspoon of sodium bicarbonate or sodium and potassium bicarbonate (in either a 3:1 or 4:1 ratio, depending on your tolerance for potassium) in 4 to 8 oz. of water. Continue taking the alkalinizing agents every hour or two until all the symptoms of overacidity have disappeared. If bingeing on highly acidic foods or beverages tends to trigger respiratory infections, also consider taking one to two dosages of colloidal silver (a natural antibacterial and anti-viral supplement) immediately following and two hours after the binge.

7

Dietary Needs for Special Groups

Specific groups such as overly acidic athletes, corporate employees and businesspeople, and children and teenagers, are at particular risk of impaired performance in their jobs or activities if particular attention is not paid to the acid-alkaline makeup of their diet. This is discussed in this section.

Athletes with Overly Acidic Constitutions

Most professional athletes must be high-alkaline producers to survive and excel in their competitive environment. However, many dedicated amateurs and weekend warriors do not have the professional athlete's buffering capability. Given the millions of Americans who regularly jog, bike, play tennis, life weights, and even compete in very strenuous events such as marathons, triathlons, and bodybuilding contests, a knowledge of your own buffering capability can give you a real edge in both enjoying and performing well in sports or athletic events.

Obviously, amateur athletes who are high-alkaline producers and have larger mineral reserves have a physiological edge on their more acidic peers. This is particularly true for those athletes who participate in strenuous anaerobic exercise, which tends to generate large amounts of lactic acid while, at the same time, depleting oxygen and the reserves of buffering substances contained within the muscles. In addition, alkaline minerals can be lost in the perspiration generated by exercise. A study published in the Annals of the New York Academy of Sciences examining mineral loss during marathon running found that athletes lost significant amounts of sodium, potassium, magnesium, and chloride; even small amounts of calcium may be lost in perspiration.

As a result, not all amateur athletes have the healthy alkaline constitution necessary to benefit from (and, in some cases, properly digest) the many protein powders, bars, and high-protein regimens that are recommended for athletic performance. In addition, overly acidic athletes may not perform as well on the highly acidic meat-based diet that is often recommended for those doing strenuous activities such as weight lifting or playing football.

Athletes who are overly acidic will probably find that they have much more energy and perform better when they eat a less acidic, more alkaline diet. They may feel better consuming vegetable-based sources of protein or fish instead of red meat. They can also benefit from the use of alkaline mineral supplements and alkalinizing agents, particularly if they are using the highly acidic glucose and protein-based powders to gain weight and/or muscle mass or are eating protein bars for additional calories and energy. In such cases, the use of alkalinizing agents one hour after ingesting these foods will help to neutralize the acid load that they produce within the body.

Corporate America

Corporate employees will enjoy better health and greater productivity if they eat according to their pH needs. Most corporations are constantly looking for ways in which they can boost productivity and limit absenteeism. Most of the solutions have focused on improving morale, creating better mental programming, and enhancing physical fitness through corporate trainings, pep talks, and elaborate corporate fitness centers. However, the importance of meal planning, based on the relative alkalinity or acidity of the employees, has been totally ignored. Many corporations now provide meals for their employees through corporate kitchens. Corporate chefs can greatly benefit the employees of the companies they work for by incorporating the principles of acid and alkaline foods into their menu planning.

Awareness of these principles can provide management with a powerful tool to greatly improve the health and productivity at all levels of the organization. The more education management can provide to all employees regarding the performance and health benefits of maintaining a slightly alkaline pH, the more the company will benefit from reduced health care costs and absenteeism. The result will be a more energetic, effective, enthusiastic, and productive workforce.

I have frequently observed the detrimental effects on energy and productivity that highly acidic food, served in corporate settings, can have on tired, overworked, and highly stressed businesspeople. Several years ago, I did a consulting job for a West Coast corporation. I was closeted, off-site, for three days of meetings with the executives of the company. Many of the participants had been traveling extensively for the previous month. They were constantly drinking highly acidic beverages laden with caffeine, such as coffee and colas, to try to boost their flagging energy.

At the meetings we were served a series of highly acidic meals and snacks. For example, at the end of one long work session, we were given Chinese takeout food for lunch, including fried pork, egg rolls, and oil-drenched noodles and rice dishes. Bowls of M&M's and chocolate cake for dessert were then left out for us to snack on for the rest of the afternoon—along with other acidic snacks such as chocolate bars, licorice sticks, cookies, and soft drinks.

I did not eat most of these dishes, preferring to eat the less acidic salad and only the cooked vegetables from the pork dish. By midafternoon, the sales manager, who had been downing coffee and chocolate candies since he had arrived the day before, turned to me and confided, "It's only two in the afternoon, and I feel horrible." This basically healthy man in his mid-forties further confided that these energy drops happened to him frequently and he had no idea why.

At another all-day strategy meeting that I attended, twelve people from various parts of the country gathered in a small conference room of a downtown hotel. Everyone began the day bright-eyed, energetic, and full of ideas. Our hosts then served us a highly acidic breakfast consisting of orange juice, ham-and-cheese omelets, hash brown potatoes, buttered toast, and a basket of sweet rolls, with plenty of strong coffee.

After a lunch of equally acidic foods, I could not help but notice that everyone's energy dropped immediately. Their formerly bright eyes became dull and glazed over. Several of the participants even developed runny noses. When the waiters offered more coffee during a midafternoon break, virtually everyone accepted this further assault on their pH-regulating systems in an effort to boost their declining energy. Only the naturally alkaline peak performers can maintain their enthusiasm and vitality at these meetings after days of eating highly acidic corporate fare.

If you are a corporate employee or business consultant and are frequently expected to attend meetings, seminars, trade shows, and conventions, you may find that eating highly acidic business fare is causing a drop in your energy and vitality. Neutralize these ill effects with a corporate survival kit. Instead of heading for the coffee, colas, and M&M's, use alkalinizing agents like sodium and potassium bicarbonate to neutralize excess acidity and restore your energy levels. In addition, taking digestive enzymes both during and after corporate meals will also help to maintain your energy level (see my book on enzymes for further details on digestive enzymes). This same tip applies to anyone who is frequently faced with eating highly acidic food at civic-related or social events.

Children and Teenagers

The consumption of an overly acidic diet by children and teenagers should be of great concern to all parents. Children and teenagers are in a crucial phase of physical growth: Their bones are still growing, and their organs are still increasing in size. Even maturation of the sexual organs does not begin until the early teens. Children need an abundant intake of alkaline minerals and other nutrients in order to develop strong muscles and bones and create the alkaline mineral reserves within their cells and tissues. For example, teenagers need 1500 mg of calcium a day to support their bone growth. This is the same amount of calcium needed by a postmenopausal woman experiencing a significant amount of bone loss who is at risk for osteoporosis.

However, a Gallup study indicated that although most children try to eat a balanced diet, few do. Half of all children do not meet the RDA for vitamin B6, calcium, and zinc (calcium is one of the critical alkaline reserve minerals). The study also found that a child who is deficient in one nutrient is probably deficient in others. The poor nutritional status of many children has been confirmed in a number of research studies.

For example, one study, published in the Journal of the American Dietetics Association, examined the diet of schoolchildren in New York State. On the day they were surveyed, 40 percent of the students did not eat vegetables, except for potatoes or tomato sauce, while 36 percent ate at least four different types of snack foods. Children of lower socioeconomic status were found to have less diversity in their diets than children of more affluent families. However, the children from more affluent families were found to eat more snack foods—snack foods in our society are invariably highly acidic.

The diet of many children and teenagers in this country is highly acidic, mainly through ignorance. Even more than adults, children tend to eat heavily promoted, low-nutrient, and highly acidic foods. The staples of the diet for many children tend to be soft drinks, candy bars, cookies, hamburgers, hot dogs, pizza, chips, French fries, milkshakes, and ice cream. Many children begin their day with a highly sugared refined-grain cereal, white toast and butter, fruit drinks, and frozen pastries or waffles. This is followed by a lunch of processed meat on white bread, potato chips, and cookies, all washed down with a highly acidic soft drink. And dinners often consist of highly acidic fast food.

This acid assault depletes the mineral reserves of children and teenagers and puts an enormous stress on their acid-buffering systems and organs of elimination even before their growth and development has been completed. As a result, there is an epidemic of illnesses related to overacidity in children and teenagers. Many children suffer from four to six respiratory ailments per year, such as colds, flus, middle-ear infections, and bronchitis. Moreover, the incidences of childhood allergies and asthma have increased dramatically over the past few decades. The incidence of asthma has doubled since 1980, making it the leading chronic disorder in children under seventeen years of age. There are now between 5 and 6 million children diagnosed with asthma. Furthermore, diabetes and cancer are seen more frequently in younger individuals.

Symptoms of overacidity are now affecting the performance of children and teenagers as well as their health. Many children find it difficult to concentrate in the classroom or while doing their homework. Attention deficit disorder is estimated to occur in 3 to 6 percent of American children. There is more violent behavior in the schools and on the streets. Children continue to succumb to cigarettes, recreational drugs, and alcohol, all of which are highly acidic substances. Parents need to educate themselves about the short- and long-term deleterious effects of children and teenagers consuming large amounts of overly acidic foods and beverages. Children have no idea about the negative consequences that eating these highly acidic foods will have on their performance capability and health once they enter adulthood.

I have treated many overly acidic and nutrient deficient children in my clinical practice- from infants to teenagers. Many of these children have suffered from frequent colds, earaches, asthma, food allergies, digestive problems, acne, eczema, hyperactivity, juvenile rheumatoid arthritis, poor mental and emotional development and a host of other health issues. Changing the diet of these children to a more alkaline, nutrient rich, allergen free diet has been very helpful in changing their pattern of ill health to one of robust health, wellness, energy and vitality.

The following are a number of tips that I have found to be helpful in working with parents and helping them to better plan their children's diets and create a state of healthy alkalinity in their children.

Probiotics are beneficial for infants and young children who are suffering from colic, diarrhea, gas and other digestive complaints. Chamomile tea is also beneficial for colic and ginger tea for nausea in children such as car sickness. These nutrients will help to reduce acidic inflammatory reactions as well as spasm.

Supplement their diets with flaxseed oil. This is even beneficial for children as little as one to two years olds who can benefit from ½ teaspoon per day. The omega 3 fatty acids contained in flaxseed oil are essential for the healthy growth and development of children. It also helps to prevent inflammatory conditions in children.

Docosahexaenoic acid (DHA), another omega 3 fatty acid, is useful for breastfeeding mothers who are vegetarians and vegans to support the growth and development of their infant through their breast milk.

Breast milk generally provides all of the nutrients that babies need up to four to six months old, except for vitamin D. 400 I.U. of vitamin D starting in the first few days of life. After that age, as babies change to a more solid diet, their iron requirement increases. Multivitamins and minerals for infants and young children may also be beneficial. One or two tablespoons of fresh, mixed vegetable juice mixed into keifer or yogurt can provide alkaline nutrient support for fussy children.

Virtually all of the food packed into children's lunch boxes and all of the treats they are given, both at school and at home, are highly acidic. Avoid giving your children lunches consisting of highly acidic pizza, hamburgers, potato chips, soft drinks, brownies, and chocolate chip cookies. Instead, provide them with garden burgers, chicken or tofu hot dogs, tuna sandwiches, baked chips, air-popped popcorn, carrot and celery sticks, and nondairy beverages or water.

Do not reward your children with candy bars, cookies, and cakes made with refined white sugar and flour. Instead, give them cookies and cakes made with non-gluten whole-grain flours and sweeteners such as xylitol, stevia, rice bran syrup and molasses that are less acid-forming. Molasses is a very rich source of many alkaline minerals, especially potassium or better yet avoid food rewards altogether.

Children with allergies should have pastries made with non-wheat flours such as rice, oat, millet, and tapioca flours. A wide variety of these products are readily available in health food stores, and they tend to be as delicious as their less healthy counterparts. I also recommend eliminating dairy products and using the many dairy substitutes made from rice, nut, soy, coconut and other sources for milk, cheese, cream cheese, sour cream and desserts. This will help to cut down on the frequency of colds, earaches, constipation, colic and other digestive complaints and skin conditions in children.

Avoid using white bread, lunch meats when making your children's lunches and other meals since they are too high in salt content. This is also true for salty chips, pretzels and popcorn, pizza and many canned soups. Try to use no salt or low salt options. Too much table salt creates overacidity in the body and is unhealthy for children and adults, both.

Children and teenagers whose performance and health are suffering because of overacidity should follow the same alkaline power diet as their parents. Overly acidic children can also benefit from the use of a vitamin and mineral supplement. Parents may also want to give their children one-quarter to one-half the normal adult dose of an alkalinizing agent such as sodium and potassium bicarbonate when they come down with common respiratory conditions. (Many teenagers are big enough to take a full adult dose.) Consult with your pediatrician or family physician if you have any questions on the advisability of doing this.

8

Restoring Your Alkaline Mineral Reserves

One of the most important ways to restore buffering capability is to replenish the body's mineral reserves. The larger the reserves of alkaline minerals contained within the body, the greater the capability a person has to neutralize the acids that result from eating acidic foods or doing strenuous exercise or that are the waste products of the body's ongoing metabolic processes. The mineral content of our cells and extracellular fluids must be maintained to enable the body to remain slightly alkaline. Our reserves of bone minerals, in particular, need to be constantly replenished since the bones provide an important reservoir of alkaline minerals that help to keep the pH of our blood stable when our other buffer systems are no longer functioning as well.

It is difficult if not impossible to replenish our mineral reserves through diet alone. The use of mineral supplements to rebuild our reserves is essential once we reach our forties and fifties. The use of supplemental minerals will allow overly acidic individuals to build up their reserves much more rapidly. In addition, our modern diet is so deficient in many of the essential major and trace minerals that it is virtually impossible to take in adequate amounts of them through food alone. This is particularly true in overly acidic individuals whose cells, tissues, and bones may be lacking many of the minerals needed for optimal health and performance.

How the Modern Diet Became Deficient In Alkaline Minerals

The alkaline mineral deficit of our modern diet is a problem of relatively recent origin. In late Paleolithic times, 35,000 to 20,000 years ago, our hunter-gatherer ancestors ate a highly varied diet that supplied all of the major minerals and most of the trace minerals. These people ate greater amounts of food than we consume today, yet their food contained more nutrients and fiber and fewer calories than the diets of most people in Western societies. Moreover, their main beverage was water, not highly acidic beverages like our soft drinks, coffee, tea, wine, and beer.

How the Development of Agriculture Changed the Food Supply

Agriculture began in various parts of the world 10,000 to 5,000 years ago as the Paleolithic hunter-gatherers made the transition to farming. While cultivation of crops is usually thought of as an advancement in human development, it actually caused the nutritional value of the human diet to decline. With the advent of farming, only certain crops were cultivated to the exclusion of others, and only certain strains within each crop were selected to be cultivated from year to year.

The human diet consequently became much more limited. A person was less likely to consume a broad range of minerals as well as other nutrients. However, in these early days, vegetables and fruits still had significant nutritional value since they were raised in naturally organic, mineral-rich soil, and according to farming practices that returned minerals to the earth.

Up to the days of our grandparents and great-grandparents, most people still lived on farms and ate fresh seasonal produce. If they lived in cities, they still ate fruits and vegetables grown locally and sold in season. These foods were still grown using farming practices that included time-tested methods such as crop rotation, mulching, and manure fertilization, which helped insure high mineral content in the crops.

How Modern Food Production Affects the Mineral Content of Foods

As the Industrial Revolution introduced mass production to agriculture, methods to refine grains and sugar were developed, and the processing of oils was soon to follow. New food products were created at the expense of nutrition, as minerals and other nutrients were removed during the manufacturing process. After World War II, farming itself changed radically.

Manufacturers of chemicals, such as the phosphates and nitrates used in wartime to produce explosives, needed new markets for their products. These chemicals became the raw materials for producing fertilizers. By 1960, 97 percent of all crops were treated with chemical fertilizers that used salt-based nitrogen, phosphorus, and potassium (NPK fertilizers). This method of growing food produced fruits and vegetables that were full of color and perfectly shaped. However, these new farming techniques sacrificed mineral content. For the last fifty years, America's farmland has been progressively stripped of minerals, notably selenium, zinc, and a variety of trace minerals.

In response to this potentially devastating loss, some farmers who are aware of the deterioration of the soil have turned to organic farming to restore their land and have produced crops of higher nutritional value. The production of organic foods is accelerating each year, far beyond early expectations; organic foods are even starting to be sold in supermarkets. A study published in the Journal of Applied Nutrition reported on over two years of research in which the nutrient content of organic produce, including potatoes, apples, peas, and corn, was measured. The results showed that the organic produce had twice the nutrient content of regular supermarket produce. Another comparison of the nutrient content of organic produce with regular supermarket produce appeared as a review article in the Townsend Letter for Doctors & Patients. Lab tests again found that organic produce contained double the amount of vitamins and minerals as standard produce. At the same time, the organic foods also contained lower amounts of toxic heavy metal residues including lead, aluminum, and mercury.

The Problem with the Standard American Diet

With the depletion of soil minerals, on the one hand, and the processing and refining of foods, on the other, the American diet is highly acidic and at the same time does not supply sufficient minerals to buffer these acids. As I discussed earlier in this book, the great majority of foods commonly eaten in our country are highly acidic—red meat, dairy products, refined flour and sugar, coffee, and soft drinks—while only a scant portion of meals are comprised of less acid, more alkaline vegetables, whole grains, legumes, starches, fish, and certain fresh fruits like papaya and melons. As mentioned in earlier in this book, a comparison of the foods eaten per person each year shows 2143 pounds of acid or acid-forming foods versus only 380 pounds of alkaline foods.

Our plant foods today have been grown in depleted and exhausted soils. In addition, many of the foods we eat have been refined and are thus stripped of their mineral content. Therefore, the alkaline minerals contained within the foods we eat are inadequate to buffer our heavy intake of protein. For example, the amounts of minerals lost when whole wheat is refined are 67 percent of the calcium, 77 percent of the magnesium, 79 percent of the potassium, 44 percent of the iron, and 62 percent of the zinc. The baked goods and fast foods we eat in great quantity also rely on processed and refined ingredients that are low in minerals.

For health, the balance between minerals such as sodium and potassium is also important. Today's methods of food processing and cooking add acidic table salt to foods and remove alkaline potassium. As a result, we consume about one and a half times more sodium chloride than potassium, with our average daily intake of sodium ranging from 2300 mg to 6900 mg. Take a look at how today's foods compare with those of our Paleolithic ancestors. An apple contains 1 mg of sodium and 301 mg of potassium, whereas a piece of apple pie contains 110 mg of sodium and 80 mg of potassium. A portion of venison, one of the game meats eaten by our early ancestors, contains 65 mg of sodium, whereas today's hot dog contains 1100 mg of sodium.

Our calcium intake has also declined. The Paleolithic diet provided 1500 to 2000 mg of calcium a day, contributed by wild plant foods, meat, and the bones of small animals and fowl. There is more calcium in wild fruits and vegetables than in cultivated hybrids. Early humans took in more than enough calcium (and iron) by modern standards. The average daily intake of calcium for Americans today is only 400 to 500 mg.

Yet while agriculture and our food supply have changed, our genes have not. Ninety-nine percent of our genes are ancient in origin, dating from our earliest prehistoric ancestors. Of the remaining 1 percent, 99 percent of these originate prior to the time that systematic growing of crops began. Thus, most of our physiology and biochemistry were adapted to dietary conditions that existed prior to 10,000 years ago—which is astounding to consider, given the way we eat today.

The Dietary Content of Alkaline Minerals and Bone Structure

The decline in the minerals and other nutrient content of the diet occurred once humans switched from the Paleolithic mode of hunter-gatherer to farming. This is quite apparent when scientists examine the skeletal remains of ancient humans. Paleolithic men and women had a body structure similar to that of modern athletes. Skeletal remains show that these people had large, dense bones and strong teeth, reflecting the huge mineral reserves they had that could be used for buffering acids in the diet. There are no structural signs of overacidity, such as osteoporosis. The hunter-gatherers were also tall. Preagricultural humans were our height or slightly taller for over a million years. Men grew to be, on average, five feet ten inches to six feet two inches, and the average height of women was five feet five.

We tend to think of our ancient ancestors as being shorter than we are. However, it was only after the advent of agriculture, 10,000 to 5,000 years ago, and the more limited array of foods that domestication of crops provided, that height declined. Our immediate historic ancestors of the past five to ten millennia were shorter than modern human beings. This point is strikingly illustrated if you visit a museum exhibiting clothes that human beings wore 500 years ago: You're likely to see small mannequins, wearing clothes that would nearly fit a child today. When people of today visit the birthplaces of great artists and historic villages, they usually have to stoop to walk through the doors that were high enough for the people of Mozart's or Shakespeare's day and for our colonial ancestors.

It is only in the last hundred years that human beings began to regain stature because of the higher fat and protein content of our diets and our higher caloric intake. Modern Americans tend to be taller and more muscular and to carry more weight than previous generations. However, because our mineral intake is so low, we have regained our former height but not the former mineral content of our bones. Unlike the dense bones of our Paleolithic ancestors, the bones of many Americans are porous and even osteoporotic. Our teeth are also weaker, resulting in widespread tooth decay and gum recession. The only exceptions tend to be the small minority of individuals who have a naturally alkaline constitution or other individuals who have made the effort to consume a mineral-rich diet.

The Acid-Alkaline Mineral Needs of Modern Humans

Human tissue contains all ninety-two elements that naturally occur on Earth. We require sodium, potassium, calcium, and phosphorus in relatively large quantities, in dosages of hundreds to thousands of milligrams per day. We also require trace amounts of many other minerals on a daily basis, such as chromium, copper, iodine, iron, selenium, and zinc. The average amounts of minerals in a 154-pound man are as follows:

Acid-Forming Elements		Alkaline-Forming Elements	
Chlorine	85 g	Sodium	63 g
Phosphorus	670 g	Potassium	150 g
Sulfur	112 g	Calcium	1160 g
Iodine	0.014 g	Magnesium	21 g
		Iron	3 g

Many people are not consuming the quantity of minerals needed to maintain these mineral reserves and normal body composition. The consequences of such deficiency are well documented. Studies of people of the South Pacific done in the 1930s found that once these people changed from their traditional diet to one that emphasized refined flour and sugar, they developed many diseases commonly found in industrialized cultures, such as diabetes, tooth decay, and even deformity of the jawbones, in just one or two generations. In our own culture, the prevalence of osteoporosis is a telling sign of just how widespread mineral depletion has become. One-third of American women will develop some form of osteoporosis, as will 10 to 15 percent of American men.

Taking a Mineral Supplement

To counteract the lack of minerals in the food we eat, most people need to supplement their diet with a variety of minerals. The optimal dose of minerals varies by individual, depending on whether the minerals are needed for maintenance or to correct a deficiency. The following chart lists alkalinizing minerals and dosages that are appropriate for a person who has a tendency to be acidic or is overly acidic. These minerals can correct a pH imbalance directly; some will also promote the chemical pathway necessary for a healthy pH. For example, chromium and manganese are necessary for the healthy metabolism of sugar, a substance that can potentially be highly acidifying to the system. Calcium can be taken in either an acid or an alkaline form: Calcium carbonate is alkaline, derived from limestone. Calcium lactate and calcium citrate are acidifying forms.

Not only will mineral supplements restore the alkaline reserves of the body, thereby improving our buffering capability, but they are also needed for the activation of hundreds of essential enzyme reactions needed for healthy metabolism, digestion, and immunity, as well as other vital functions. Having sufficient levels of minerals within the body helps support our physical energy and stamina and helps us to recover rapidly from physical and mental exertion.

Mineral Supplement Dosage per Day

Mineral	Daily Dose
Calcium	800–1500 mg
Magnesium	400–800 mg
Potassium	99–300 mg
Zinc	15–30 mg
Manganese	5-10 mg
Chromium	200 mcg
Iron*	10–18 mg
Selenium	50–200 mcg
Copper	1–2 mg
Iodine	150–225 mcg
Boron	3 mg

*Men should consider taking multi-mineral formulas without added iron because of possible toxicity since men do not lose iron, as women do, through menstruation. Many postmenopausal women may have low iron stores, particularly if they suffer from iron-deficiency anemia during their active reproductive years. These women may benefit from continued moderate iron supplementation until the deficiency is corrected, at which point they should switch to an iron-free supplement.

It is important to read the label carefully before buying a mineral product for use in an alkalinity restoration program. Many products that are labeled high-potency vitamin and mineral combinations tend to have higher dosages of vitamins than minerals. This is particularly true of formulations of one to two tablets or capsules per day. It is very difficult to incorporate the amount of supplemental minerals that an overly acidic person needs in so few tablets or capsules.

I instead recommend buying separate vitamin and high-potency mineral supplements to insure that dosage levels of the minerals are in the therapeutic ranges. This will usually require at least three to four tablets or capsules a day for a multi-nutrient product. Individual minerals can also be purchased separately.

9

Using Alkalinizing Agents for Quick Symptom Relief

Alkalinizing agents can be tremendously beneficial in assisting the body to rapidly neutralize overacidity. Alkalinizing agents such as sodium and potassium bicarbonate, sodium and potassium citrate, and sodium phosphate can relieve the symptoms of overacidity within a very short time. Alkalinizing agents can rapidly catalyze a shift from overacidity to a healthier alkaline state. The almost immediate relief that these agents can provide makes them an extremely powerful part of any program in which an individual needs to restore their buffering capability for both peak performance and optimal health.

Two other alkalinizing agents, buffered vitamin C and alkaline water, are also tremendously beneficial and should and can be used daily as part of an alkalinity restoration program. They are not only powerful buffering agents, but will also help to build up your mineral reserves. In addition, they both have powerful antioxidant effects, helping to protect the body from heart attacks, strokes, and immune-system problems. While a less acid, more alkaline diet and the use of supplemental alkaline minerals will begin to restore our buffering capability; these remedies tend to work slowly and will not provide the quick symptom relief seen with the use of alkalinizing agents. In this section I also discuss two other alkalinizing treatments: alkaline water and magnetic therapy. Supplemental oxygen therapy, which is an extremely powerful alkalinizing therapy, is covered in depth in my book on this topic.

It is important to realize that the need for alkalinizing agents can vary greatly with one's level of health, as well as one's current levels of environmental, dietary, and emotional stress. For example, when one is trying to recover from an acute illness or is eating a highly acidic diet, the need for alkalinizing agents is much greater and dosages may be larger and taken more frequently. In contrast, during periods of good health, relative lack of emotional stress, or eating a more alkaline diet, the need for alkalinizing agents may decline to smaller dosages taken once or twice a day for maintenance purposes.

For example, when you have a severe cold, you might need as much as one-half to one full teaspoon of a sodium bicarbonate or a sodium and potassium bicarbonate combination, taken three to four times a day, to effectively reduce symptoms. However, when you are symptom-free and feeling well, you may only need half a teaspoon once or twice a day. (These dosages, of course, may vary according to the needs of each individual.)

Sodium Bicarbonate

Sodium bicarbonate is a nontoxic, white crystalline powder that has a mild, neutral taste. It is also referred to as baking soda and bicarbonate of soda. As a buffering agent, sodium bicarbonate easily reacts with other compounds, making acidic substances more alkaline and alkaline substances more acidic. Sodium bicarbonate produces a significantly alkaline end product with a pH of 8.1.

Not only is sodium bicarbonate an essential part of the buffer system of our body, it is also active in the natural ecology of the Earth. Sodium bicarbonate plays a role in maintaining the pH balance in all living things. It is found in lake sediments, mineral deposits, groundwater, and even the ocean, where it helps stabilize the amount of carbon dioxide in the atmosphere.

Because of sodium bicarbonate's ability to buffer a wide variety of substances, it has many common uses within the home. People often store an opened box of sodium bicarbonate in the refrigerator as a deodorant, because it chemically neutralizes unpleasant odors which are usually caused by a strong acid, such as sour milk, or a strong alkaline food, such as spoiled fish.

Sodium bicarbonate also works as a cleanser, alkalinizing the fatty acids in dirt and grease so that they become water soluble and can be washed away. And as a leavening agent, sodium bicarbonate, or baking soda, causes baked goods to rise. It is added to dough, along with an acid such as lemon juice, and when the dough is baked, heated bubbles of carbon dioxide are released. The bubbles, trapped inside the dough, cause it to stretch and rise. Baking powder, which is also used for leavening, is a mixture of sodium bicarbonate and an acid, such as cream of tartar.

If you are concerned about your sodium intake because of high blood pressure or a history of congestive heart failure, you may want to use a combination of sodium and potassium bicarbonate instead.

Potassium Bicarbonate

Unlike sodium bicarbonate, potassium bicarbonate is only available from a chemical supply house; it is also occasionally found in nutritional supplement products. A pharmacist can also prepare a mixture of sodium bicarbonate and potassium bicarbonate, or an individual can make his or her own mixture. Like sodium bicarbonate, potassium bicarbonate is a white, crystalline, nontoxic powder. Both substances will last indefinitely if stored in a cool, dry place. However, while sodium bicarbonate has a mild, pleasant taste, potassium bicarbonate is somewhat sharp and chalky on the tongue. Potassium bicarbonate is rarely taken alone because of its unpalatable taste. It can also be irritating to the digestive tract in individuals with intestinal conditions like inflammatory small bowel disease. Furthermore, if taken alone in a high dosage for prolonged periods of time, it may cause an irregular heartbeat.

Sodium and Potassium Bicarbonate Combinations

You may find it preferable to use sodium and potassium in combination in a ratio of 3:1 to 4:1 sodium to potassium (depending on your tolerance for potassium) rather than using sodium bicarbonate alone. First of all, the digestive juices produced by the pancreas contain both sodium and potassium. In addition, many individuals do not eat enough potassium-rich foods in their diet. There are also other health benefits to supplementing with both buffering agents since this helps to maintain the sodium-potassium balance of the cells.

For a cell to be healthy there must be a predominance of potassium inside the cell and sodium outside it. This condition generates an electrical charge that allows the cell wall to control which substances enter the cell and to discharge toxins from the cell. Since the standard American diet contains an overabundance of sodium and is low in potassium (commonly supplied by fresh plant foods) our diet itself can potentially disturb the important balance of these intracellular and extracellular minerals.

While most overly acidic people tolerate sodium bicarbonate very well, using large amounts of sodium bicarbonate alone as a buffering agent is not recommended for people on a low-sodium diet, such as individuals with severe hypertension or congestive heart failure, persons taking certain heart medications, and women who are pregnant. However, there are individuals who do find potassium bicarbonate irritating to their digestive tract or have a preexisting health condition for which the use of a potassium-based supplement is contraindicated. Such individuals can use sodium bicarbonate alone as an alkalinizing agent. See your physician if you have any specific questions.

Sodium and Potassium Bicarbonate Treatments for Performance and Health

Individuals who use sodium and potassium bicarbonate for a variety of performance- or health-related reasons will vary greatly in both the dosage and the frequency with which these alkalinizing agents should be used. For instance, a person with a severe allergic reaction or an intense bout of the flu may need to use an alkalinizing agent every few hours for a short period of time until their symptoms start to diminish. At this point, dosages can be spread out to every three to four hours while the person is still in the acute phase of the illness.

In contrast, an individual with mild sinusitis may find that using bicarbonate once or twice a day on a daily basis provides enough buffering to prevent their symptoms from occurring. However, a generally recommended dosage is one-half teaspoon of a mixture of sodium bicarbonate and potassium bicarbonate in a 3:1 or 4:1 ratio (depending on how well the individual tolerates potassium). Sodium bicarbonate may be used by itself in individuals with digestive problems who find potassium supplements irritating to the intestinal tract.

Occasionally, an individual will find that he or she needs to go as high as a one-teaspoon dosage for a very short period of time in order to relieve their symptoms. Conversely, very sensitive individuals may find that a tiny dose, such as one-eighth teaspoon, is sufficient.

Physicians who work with nutritional programs to restore acid-alkaline balance often find that highly acidic people may need to use sodium and potassium bicarbonate on a regular basis, for as long as several years. Higher dosages may be necessary during the first four to six months of treatment to counteract their overacidity. The dosages can gradually be reduced, except during periods of great physical or emotional stress, when higher dosages may be necessary. At the same time, however, these physicians will place their patients on more alkalinizing diets and mineral supplementation, both of which are needed to build up the alkaline reserves of the body and counteract overacidity.

The use of alkalinizing agents alone on a long-term basis will not produce maximum therapeutic benefits unless these other restorative steps are followed so that the healthful, slightly alkaline pH of the body can be restored. However, in order to restore major body systems that are greatly overly acidic and to offset the overacidity that develops as part of the normal aging process, an individual (particularly if past midlife) may have to continue a maintenance program for a prolonged period of time or even indefinitely.

It is always helpful to begin any program to restore your acid-alkaline balance with the help of either a physician who is knowledgeable about nutritional medicine or a well-trained nutritionist.

Work-Related Physical and Mental Fatigue

Strenuous work demands and long hours can significantly increase the production of acidic waste products within the body. Using alkalinizing agents can neutralize these waste products and restore one's energy and stamina.

SUGGESTED DOSAGE: To treat physical and mental strain and fatigue, take one-half to one teaspoon of sodium bicarbonate, or a mixture of sodium bicarbonate and potassium bicarbonate in a ratio of 3:1 to 4:1 (less potassium if you tolerate it poorly), up to three times a day.

Athletic Activity

Weekend warriors and individuals who frequently participate in sports and athletic activities can also benefit from supplementing their diet with sodium bicarbonate. It can be used prophylactically to prevent muscle fatigue and to promote the healing of most athletic injuries once they have occurred. Sodium bicarbonate is also beneficial in reducing nasal congestion and a runny nose, which can result when a person has over trained or pushed their limits of endurance in such sports as long-distance running or cycling.

SUGGESTED DOSAGE: To counteract these symptoms, take one-half to one teaspoon of sodium bicarbonate, or a mixture of sodium bicarbonate and potassium bicarbonate in a ratio of 3:1 to 4:1 (less potassium if you tolerate it poorly), as often as necessary to eliminate symptoms. Cases of severe muscle spasm or an acute condition of nasal congestion may require several doses over a few hours

Colds, Flus, Sore Throats, Bronchitis, Middle-Ear Infections, Sinusitis, and Allergies

Most individuals who develop minor respiratory illnesses tend to be overly acidic (except for a small minority of the population who develop respiratory symptoms because of low enzyme production, poor detoxification, or poor oxygenation). For most people with these symptoms, restoring your body rapidly to a more healthful, slightly alkaline state is one of the most important steps that you can take to recover rapidly.

SUGGESTED DOSAGE: To treat a respiratory ailment in the acute stage (from the first sign or symptom), take one-half teaspoon of sodium bicarbonate, or a mixture of sodium bicarbonate and potassium bicarbonate in a ratio of 3:1 to 4:1 (less potassium if you tolerate it poorly), every few hours, up to 4 doses until symptoms begin to abate. Alternatively, you can take one dose before bed and another on rising in the morning. Acids tend to accumulate during the night, and a person with relatively few symptoms the night before may wake the next day with a return of their congestion. Also see my book on enzymes for additional anti-inflammatory suggestions.

In the acute stages of a respiratory infection, it's a good idea to prepare a solution of sodium bicarbonate and water in a closed container and keep it next to the bed so that you can occasionally sip on it. This constant drinking of the mixture will allow for the continuous alkalinizing of the body that is necessary to restore the environment needed for the body to control and eliminate the bacteria or viruses that are causing the symptoms. Also, be sure to continue the alkalinizing process for several days after the acute symptoms have subsided to prevent a recurrence of your symptoms.

Digestive Problems

Sodium bicarbonate is an effective buffering agent, alleviating acid indigestion, sour stomach, and heartburn. It also aids digestion by raising the pH necessary to activate the pancreatic enzymes responsible for breaking down protein. Bicarbonate can be combined with enzyme therapy to enhance the digestive process. Many people who are experiencing digestive problems have a pancreas that is producing only low amounts of bicarbonate and pancreatic enzymes. This use of digestive enzymes is discussed in detail my book on enzymes.

When combining enzymes and sodium bicarbonate, take the enzymes with the meal or immediately following it. However, sodium bicarbonate should not be taken at this time as it will interfere with the acid stage of digestion. Take sodium bicarbonate either one-half hour before a meal or one to one and one-half hours after eating, especially following a large meal. Enzymes can again be taken at this time.

SUGGESTED DOSAGE: For indigestion, take one-half teaspoon sodium bicarbonate in a half glass of water. Usually one or two doses will be sufficient taken every few hours. Sodium citrate is also effective as an antacid for indigestion.

Inflammatory Conditions

People with chronic inflammatory conditions such as food allergies, arthritis, colitis, and thyroiditis can benefit from alkalinizing with sodium bicarbonate, as it can have an anti-inflammatory effect when used over a long period of time.

SUGGESTED DOSAGE: Take one-half to one teaspoon three times per day. Preferably one half hour before a meal or two hours after a meal.

Steroid medications like prednisone are used to treat various acute and chronic inflammatory conditions. Steroid medication can only remain active in an alkaline pH. Individuals who are being treated with any cortisone-like drugs might want to consider using sodium and potassium bicarbonate to create an internal environment in which these drugs can provide the most efficacious results. Of course, consult with your own physician to discuss the advisability of doing this in your own personal case.

Cancer

Certain cancer treatment regimens also factor in a person's chemical makeup and pH. To pursue this approach to cancer treatment, it is important that a patient be assessed by a physician skilled in identifying these metabolic types and designing a corresponding regimen. Many people with cancer tend to be overly acidic and can benefit from an alkalinizing program. Such programs can include oxygen therapies and bicarbonate, both of which are potent alkalinizing agents, as well as the use of digestive enzymes. See my oxygen therapies and digestive enzymes books in regard to alternative therapies for cancer.

Osteoporosis

Sodium and potassium bicarbonate can also be used in the treatment of osteoporosis, a condition in which loss of bone density can lead to hip, vertebral, and wrist fractures. Osteoporosis is commonly seen in postmenopausal women and, less frequently, in older men. Since it is due, in part, to overacidity of the body, the use of alkalinizing agents can be an important part of the treatment program (as well as following a less acidic, more alkaline diet and supplementing with alkaline minerals like calcium and magnesium as well as vitamin D).

SUGGESTED DOSAGE: For long-term prevention and treatment, take from one-half teaspoon of sodium bicarbonate or a mixture of sodium bicarbonate and potassium bicarbonate in a ratio of 3:1 to 4:1 (depending on your tolerance for potassium) twice a day, in the morning on rising and before bedtime.

Skin Conditions

Many skin conditions, such as poison oak, poison ivy, and skin abrasions, can be ameliorated through the use of sodium bicarbonate. Fill a bathtub with tepid water and add one cup of baking soda. Take a bath in this water for as long as it is comfortable to do so. The same treatment can be used for insect bites: The alkalinizing action of the bicarbonate neutralizes the venom from the bites, reducing redness and itching.

First aid for burns. To help prevent blisters, use a cloth dipped in a solution of baking soda and ice water and apply this to the skin until all heat has gone from the burn area.

First aid for sunburn. Combine one-quarter cup baking soda with one-half cup cornstarch and add this mixture to a bath of tepid water. Soak in this as long and as often as possible.

Dental Problems

Tooth decay occurs when bacteria in the mouth digest sugars consumed in food. The end product is an acid that can begin to erode the protective outer enamel layer of the teeth. When baking soda is used to clean the teeth, it neutralizes the acid and prevents decay. The slightly abrasive texture of sodium bicarbonate also removes plaque. And when baking soda is combined with hydrogen peroxide, which has an effervescence, the bubbles also help float away food particles as well as kill bacteria in the mouth. To clean the teeth in this fashion, first dip a toothbrush in hydrogen peroxide and then in sodium bicarbonate.

Overdosing With Sodium or Potassium Bicarbonate

Overdosing with sodium and potassium bicarbonate can cause an individual to become too alkaline, a condition called alkalosis. Alkalosis can result in symptoms like tingling in the extremities and lips, as well as feeling anxious or panicked. In cases of severe overdosing, the nerves becoming overexcited, firing automatically and repeatedly. This can result in muscle spasms (tetany), which usually start in the forearms and can spread throughout the body. Tetany of the muscles involved in breathing can be fatal. In some people, bicarbonate can also cause digestive symptoms such as bloating or gas.

If any of these problems arise, immediately reduce the dosage and frequency of use. Drinking black coffee, black tea, the juice of a half lemon diluted in water, or cola drinks or taking vigorous exercise will all cause the body to become more acidic and help restore the pH to normal. Above all, be aware of which dosage regimen works best for you. If you are extremely sensitive, start with a lower dose than recommended. If you are highly acidic, you may have to use a higher dosage to obtain symptom relief.

Six to eight percent of the population is naturally alkaline and should avoid the use of alkalinizing agents altogether. If you fit this profile, the use of bicarbonate can cause you to become even more alkaline. This can result in fatigue, feelings of anxiety or panic, digestive symptoms such as gas and bloating, or tingling of the extremities, or even the more severe symptoms of alkalosis.

Sodium and Potassium Citrate

Both sodium citrate and potassium citrate are used in the treatment of a variety of kidney and bladder diseases. Sodium citrate helps relieve bacterial cystitis and interstitial (inflammatory) cystitis, while potassium citrate is especially useful for treating kidney stones. Sodium and potassium citrate alkalinize the urine and help to maintain a higher urinary pH over the long term, without alkalinizing the entire body. Sodium citrate is more often prescribed for indigestion. Sodium citrate is mild and pleasant tasting and much more easily tolerated than potassium citrate, which can sometimes cause digestive upset.

Both sodium citrate and potassium citrate can be ordered from health food stores. They are also prescribed by physicians treating kidney and bladder-related problems. Citrate is combined in nutritional products to produce magnesium citrate, calcium citrate, and various other mineral combinations.

Bacterial Cystitis

While bacterial cystitis is normally treated by antibiotics, the use of alkalinizing agents, like sodium citrate, may be helpful in reducing the symptoms of this condition.

SUGGESTED DOSAGE: 4 g of sodium citrate, taken three times a day, for at least two days to one week (4 g is the equivalent of 1/7 oz.).

Interstitial Cystitis

The symptoms of this painful and chronic inflammatory condition can be greatly improved by the use of alkalinizing agents. Sodium citrate can be used to treat interstitial cystitis in combination with sodium bicarbonate.

SUGGESTED DOSAGE: Sodium bicarbonate can be used to provide rapid relief during the acute, symptomatic phase in dosages of one-half to one teaspoon up to 2 - 4 times a day between meals until symptoms abate. Symptom relief can then be sustained with the use of the slower-acting sodium citrate in a dosage of one-half to three-quarters teaspoon twice a day.

Kidney Stones

To prevent the recurrence of acidic types of kidney stones, physicians will use potassium citrate alone or in combination with magnesium. Magnesium is added to some regimens to reduce the gastrointestinal distress caused by the use of potassium citrate alone. This regimen should be done only under a physician's care. Potassium citrate is also used in certain protocols for treating gout and more serious kidney diseases.

Digestion

Sodium citrate is effective as an antacid for indigestion. Take 4 to 8 g of sodium citrate as a single dose (this is equivalent to 1/7 to 2/7 oz.). It is important to wait at least one to one and one-half hours after eating before treatment to allow the acid phase of digestion to proceed normally.

Side Effects and Cautions When Using Sodium and Potassium Citrate

Sodium citrate is not recommended for people on a sodium-restricted diet or for those taking aluminum-based antacids. Side effects of overdosing with sodium citrate are nausea, vomiting, diarrhea, and convulsions.

Potassium citrate should be avoided by individuals with certain health problems such as urinary-tract infection, diabetes mellitus, kidney failure, adrenal insufficiency, and acute dehydration. High levels of potassium can cause tingling in the hands and feet and, in extreme cases, mental confusion, paralysis, and even cardiac arrest. Potassium citrate is also not recommended for pregnant women and nursing mothers.

Potassium citrate is generally well tolerated, although it can cause digestive symptoms such as diarrhea, abdominal discomfort, nausea, and vomiting.

Sodium Phosphate

Phosphorus is the second most abundant mineral in the body and is found in every cell. It is an easily absorbed mineral. The phosphorus compound sodium phosphate is an effective buffering agent used as an aid to improve sports performance. A typical dosage used in studies is 4g a day for three days prior to an event. This has been found to improve both anaerobic and endurance exercise. Sodium phosphate is nontoxic in normal amounts. However, taking large doses can lead to calcium loss as phosphorus interacts with calcium during metabolism.

The sodium and potassium bicarbonate described earlier in this book have an immediate alkalinizing effect on your body. However, for additional, continuous alkaline support throughout the day, I also recommend using a product called Acid Check, which is released into your body more gradually. It is a mixture containing potassium, magnesium, and calcium that comes in granular and caplet form. I recommend 2 to 3 caplets per day or if you prefer granules mix 1/4 teaspoon into 4-8 ounces of water two times a day between meals. The granular form comes in a shaker bottle, so you can also use it on the spot to neutralize highly acidic foods such as tomatoes, citrus fruits and juices, berries, salad dressings, spicy foods, sugary foods, and wine.

The granules do not alter the flavor or aroma of foods or beverages it's sprinkled but it may make them taste sweeter due to the reduced acid content. Consider keeping a bottle with you for restaurant meals, special occasions, and other times when you don't have as much control over what you eat and need to reduce the meal acidity by as much as 90%. You can purchase Acid Check at www.acidcheck.com.

Buffered Vitamin C

Almost all animals are able to produce vitamin C within their own bodies, primarily in the liver. Exceptions include guinea pigs, monkeys, and human beings. Human beings lack the enzyme necessary for the conversion of glucose to vitamin C. It is estimated that if our body were able to manufacture vitamin C, we would produce as much as 10g a day. However, the current RDA for vitamin C is a modest 60 mg.

As we are unable to produce vitamin C, we must depend on food and nutritional supplements for our supply. Many fruits and vegetables are rich sources of natural vitamin C including citrus fruits, strawberries, papayas, red and green peppers, broccoli, Brussels sprouts, tomatoes, asparagus, parsley, dark leafy greens, and cabbage. There is almost no vitamin C in meats, seeds, grains, and beans. However, when seeds, grains, and beans are sprouted, they become an excellent source of vitamin C. Unfortunately, many people eat diets that are very low in this important nutrient due to a high intake of fast and processed food.

Vitamin C is crucial for the maintenance of optimal health. While most people think of taking vitamin C when they have a cold, this remarkable vitamin has great value far beyond its use as a home remedy for nasal congestion. It has been studied for its usefulness as an antioxidant in the prevention of heart disease. Researchers have also investigated how vitamin C bolsters immune function. It has been found to activate neutrophils, which are part of the immune system's first line of defense. Vitamin C may also increase production of lymphocytes. These white cells are important in the production of antibodies and help coordinate the body's immune response to bacteria and viruses. Vitamin C may also decrease histamine production, thereby reducing the likelihood of an allergic reaction.

Millions of people use vitamin C on a daily basis for its health benefits. However, in choosing a vitamin C supplement, you must consider its effect on pH, especially when using it in high dosages, more than 1 to 2 g a day. Such dosages are commonly taken by many individuals for both treatment and prevention of many diseases. Dosages as high as 3 to 5 g per day are often used when fighting acute illnesses. Vitamin C in its natural form, ascorbic acid, is actually a mild acid.

In addition, many of the vitamin C products on the market are acid-based. This acidic form of vitamin C is fine for people who are fundamentally alkaline or have good buffering capability. However, the people who can benefit most from vitamin C tend to be overly acidic. These people need to take vitamin C in its buffered form, which is combined with alkaline minerals that increase its pH, creating a more alkaline and better tolerated form of this vitamin. Overly acidic individuals do not usually have the buffering capability to neutralize large amounts of ascorbic acid. Another benefit of using buffered vitamin C is that it is less likely to cause diarrhea or intestinal irritation, which can occur with ascorbic acid.

With buffered vitamin C, ascorbic acid is usually combined with minerals such as calcium, magnesium, potassium, and zinc. Taking calcium ascorbate alone requires supplementing with additional magnesium to keep these two minerals in balance within the body. For persons predisposed to kidney stones, taking magnesium also helps to keep the calcium soluble, so that it does not form calcium oxalate stones.

Ascorbic acid is also helpful for people who are naturally alkaline. They are able to buffer its acidity without any problem, and may even need it to balance their pH. Vitamin C is as effective at lowering pH as a cola or a cup of coffee but without the harmful effects of the caffeine or other chemicals in these beverages. Alkaline individuals often need the antioxidant effects that this vitamin provides. Since alkaline types can easily digest rich meals full of fat and protein, they also run the risk of developing heart disease caused by this diet. As an antioxidant, vitamin C can help reduce the amount of oxidized low-density lipoprotein (LDL) cholesterol in the arteries, the type of cholesterol most associated with the development of heart disease.

Alkaline Water

Several devices use an innovative technology to convert ordinary tap water, through filtration and electrolysis, into an alkaline water that has extraordinary health benefits. The technology was developed in Japan in the early 1950s; commercial devices have been available there since 1958. The equipment is extremely popular in Japan, where it has received governmental approval and sells over a million units a year.

The commercial alkaline water device fits on the countertop near the sink so it can use tap water as its source. The unit, which is slightly taller and thicker than a large dictionary on end, is an electrical appliance connected to the kitchen faucet to perform electrolysis on tap water before you drink it or use it for cooking or cleaning. When the tap water enters the unit, it is first filtered to remove all chlorine, impurities, odors, and tastes. Next, the water passes into an electrolysis chamber equipped with positive and negative electrodes. Positive ions are attracted to negative electrodes, which creates water with an excess amount of electrons, thereby raising the pH of the water to levels as high as 9 to 11. This highly alkaline water is diverted into a stream that comes out the faucet to be used for drinking and cooking.

In contrast, negative ions are attracted to the positive electrode in the chamber. Through electrolysis, this water gains a positive charge and becomes more acidic, with its pH decreasing to 4 or less. This acid water is diverted into a separate hose that sits in the sink and can be used for washing hands, cleaning fruits and vegetables, sterilizing cutting boards or kitchen utensils, skin care, and treating minor wounds.

The benefits of the alkaline water created through electrolysis far exceed just its ability to gently raise the pH of the cells and tissues of the body and to neutralize acids. Because the alkaline water has gained a significant number of free electrons through the electrolysis process, it is able to donate these electrons to active oxygen radicals in the body, thereby becoming a super antioxidant. By donating its excess free electrons, alkaline water is able to block the oxidation of normal tissue by free oxygen radicals.

Another significant benefit of the electrolysis process is that the cluster size of the alkaline water is reduced by about 50 percent from the cluster size of tap water. This allows the ionized alkaline water to be much more readily absorbed by the body, thereby increasing the water's hydrating ability and its ability to carry its negative ions and alkalinizing effect to all the cells and tissues of the body. If you are overly acidic, an alkaline water device can provide a safe, gentle, and effective way of restoring the pH balance of all the cells in your body as well as providing excess free electrons to act as super antioxidants. For more information on alkaline water devices, see the appendix.

Drinking four to six glasses of alkaline water a day will help to neutralize overacidity and over time will help to restore your buffering capability. Alkaline water should also be used when conditions of overacidity develop, such as a cold, the flu or bronchitis. Like vitamins C, E, and beta-carotene, the alkaline water acts as an antioxidant because of its excess supply of free electrons. This can help to protect the body against the development of heart disease, strokes, immune dysfunctions, and other common ailments.

Because acid water is mildly astringent, it can be used to restore the protective mantle of the skin, which is naturally acid. Over time, washing the skin with acid water has cosmetic benefits, improving the texture and quality of the skin. Because of the small cluster size of the water molecules, the water is able to hydrate the outer layer of the skin much more effectively than ordinary tap or bottled water. CAUTION: Acid water is intended for external use only and it should never be ingested.

Magnets

Modern research has found that magnetic therapy has a profound healing effect on a variety of medical conditions including pain, spasms, bone fractures, neurological conditions, and depression. Therapeutic magnets create these benefits, in part, by producing alkalinizing effects on cells and tissues.

Magnets come in two types, the static or permanent magnet, such as the ones found sticking to many household refrigerators, and electromagnets, whose field is created by running an electrical current through a coil. Magnetic field strength is measured in gauss. The Earth has its own magnetic field, measuring less than 10 gauss, while magnets used for recreational and therapeutic use will have gauss ranging from 300 to 4000. Magnetic fields used for medical diagnostic procedures such as magnetic resonance imaging (MRI) will have gauss in excess of 10,000.

Magnets used in therapeutic applications come in various shapes and sizes from as small as one-half inch in diameter to six-inch squares. When larger areas of the body require treatment, smaller magnets are often sewn into a fabric, thereby creating a seat cushion or full-body mattress. While magnets were originally made from iron ore, most of today's commercially available magnets are ceramic. They are permanent and hold their gauss for decades.

Magnets have been used for many medical applications. The primary uses have been to relieve pain from soft-tissue injuries such as sprains, strains, bruises, bursitis, tendonitis, arthritis, and lower back pain, and to facilitate wound healing. Magnets have also been used for treating depression and migraine headaches and for shortening recovery times from physical exertion. Interestingly, the FDA has approved the application of electromagnetic fields to broken bones that have failed to heal. The electrical coil is placed around the break and left on for up to two to three months. This treatment has proved quite successful in uniting and healing broken bones.

Recently, interest in the therapeutic use of magnetic fields has increased dramatically because of their use in sports medicine and through double-blind research studies. Magnets are now available for soft-tissue injuries of the ankle, knee, wrist, elbow, and shoulders.

Several scientific studies have confirmed anecdotal evidence about the therapeutic benefits of magnetic field stimulation and prompting a number of new studies. The first study, reported in the Archives of Physical Medicine and Rehabilitation, was a double-blind study designed to test the effect of magnets on fifty patients suffering from pain associated with post-polio syndrome. All patients were told to hold the active magnets or inactive devices over the area of most intense pain for forty-five minutes. Prior to the treatment, the patients were asked to rate their pain on a scale of 1 (no pain) to 10 (extreme pain). After the treatment, the patients were again asked to rate their pain. The twenty-nine who used active magnets reported a reduction in pain from 9.6 to 4.4; the twenty-one who used the placebo device reported a much smaller decline, from 9.5 to 8.4.

The second study, reported in the Australia New Zealand Journal of Psychiatry, exposed seventeen patients suffering from depression to an electromagnetic field for five daily sessions. Eleven of the seventeen patients showed a marked improvement that lasted for two weeks after the treatments, with no reported adverse effects.

A third double-blind study, published in the American Journal of Pain Management, reported that the wearing of magnet-laden socks seemed to reduce or eliminate the pain associated with a foot disorder common in diabetics. The constant wearing of magnetic devices dramatically suppressed the neuropathic symptoms of burning pain, numbness, and tingling in diabetic patients' feet. Diabetic peripheral neuropathy is a progressive deterioration of nerve function in the extremities that can trigger pain in the feet. It is notoriously difficult to treat, and often the patient becomes disabled.

The study involved nineteen patients suffering from foot pain, ten of whom were diabetic. All participants wore special "magnet socks" for four months. Real magnets were sewn into one foot of each of the pair of socks, while the other foot contained a fake magnet (the placebo). Patients were not told which sock contained the real magnet, and socks were switched from one foot to the other after the first month of the study. At the end of four months, 90 percent of the diabetic subjects reported a dramatic reduction in foot pain. In contrast, just one third of the nondiabetic patients reported symptom reduction after magnetic therapy. The results of this study show the effects of the magnetic therapy to be palliative but not curative, since symptoms recur when the magnet is removed.

The exact mechanism of action for the therapeutic use of magnetic fields is unknown. There are, however, several theories of how magnets may provide therapeutic benefits, and it is possible that two or more of the suspected mechanisms may be operating simultaneously. The first theory is that magnetic fields increase blood flow to the area exposed to the field. This allows for increased oxygen and nutrients to enter the area and for waste products to be removed more rapidly, thus decreasing inflammation and relieving pain.

A second theory is that the magnetic field may affect pain receptors. It produces a slight anesthetic effect by altering neurochemical levels in the brain, including dopamine, monamines, and serotonin. These are the same neurochemicals that are related to depression and chronic pain when their production is diminished. This theory also suggests that magnetic fields may actually increase the production of endorphins, chemicals that act as natural pain relievers. A third theory is that the negative, or north pole, of a static magnetic field increases the level of alkalinity in the cells and thereby reduces the level of cellular acidity, inflammation, and pain. Thus the use of the negative pole of a magnet helps to restore the body's naturally slightly alkaline state.

The major proponent of the alkalinizing effect of the negative pole of a magnetic field was William H. Philpott, MD, a psychiatrist who researched and wrote extensively on this subject. Philpott, who won the Linus Pauling Award from the Orthomolecular Health Society in 1998, spent years researching and observing the beneficial effects of the negative pole of a magnetic field on various medical conditions. Philpott concluded that the negative or north pole of a magnetic field is life enhancing and promotes health. He stated that the magnetic field generated by the north magnetic pole increases cellular alkalinity, activates the enzymes that process free radicals, and frees oxygen from its bound state in free radicals, thereby increasing the production of ATP in cells.

As a result of these biochemical changes, the negative magnetic field speeds healing, reduces cellular stress, increases the production of melatonin (thereby aiding sleep), and assists in fighting bacteria, viruses, and even cancer. Philpott has found these negative-pole magnets effective for such varied conditions as chronic pain, inflammation, arthritis, diabetes, depression and other mental conditions, addictions, movement disorders, pelvic and intestinal disorders, and eye problems. For people who are overly acidic, these negative-pole magnets may assist in restoring and maintaining the natural slightly alkaline balance the body needs for optimal performance and health.

Magnets with a negative pole on one side are available in a variety of sizes, shapes, and gauss strengths, and as mattress pads and seat cushions. I personally favor the use of negative pole magnets over positive or neutral magnets.

Oxygen Therapies

Oxygen is the most abundant element found within our bodies and has a profound effect upon our body chemistry. Individuals who develop health conditions like respiratory illnesses, hardening of the arteries, and iron deficiency anemia may become overly acidic because of decreased oxygenation of their cells and tissues. The use of oxygen therapies can help to reduce acidosis and promotes a more healthy alkaline state within the body. See my book on oxygen therapies for more information on the subject.

10

The Role of a Healthy Lifestyle

Overly acidic individuals need to carefully assess their habits when undertaking a program to restore their body to a more naturally healthy alkaline pH. Emotional and mental stress, a hectic, fast-paced lifestyle, and hard physical exercise will tend to generate acidic waste products within the body. All of these factors increase the wear and tear on our buffer systems as well as the lungs and kidneys, our main organs of elimination. Many studies have confirmed that stress does, indeed, accelerate the aging of the body and plays a significant role in the development of disease. In contrast, by practicing stress modification through leading a calmer and more peaceful life and engaging in moderate aerobic physical activity, you can actually improve circulation and oxygenation to all of the tissues and organs within the body. Over time, our buffering capability and the health of our organs of elimination can actually improve with these healthful practices.

Physical Exercise

Overly acidic people tend to feel their best when engaged in aerobic activity that is moderately strenuous and can be done in a relaxed and leisurely way. Activities in this category include golf, swimming, walking, and bicycling at a leisurely pace. With these types of exercise, a person will tend to breathe more deeply and slowly. Over time, this helps to improve the elasticity of our lungs and relaxes the diaphragm and chest muscles, thereby allowing us to inhale more oxygen.

Moderate aerobic exercise also relaxes, dilates, and expands the network of blood vessels in the body, and enables the heart to work more efficiently.

With improved circulation, the alkalinizing oxygen that we breathe in is better able to reach all of our tissues and organs, promoting a more alkaline pH throughout the body. Better circulation and oxygenation improve the health of all our organs, including our pH-regulating organs such as the lungs and kidneys. Acidic waste products such as carbon dioxide are more effectively removed from the cells via exhalation and through the urinary tract. Moderate aerobic exercise also produces less lactic acid and is less likely to deplete the level of oxygen and buffering substances within the muscles than more strenuous physical activities like long-distance running or weight lifting.

Stress Management

Emotional and mental stress generates acidic waste products within the body that can put undue wear and tear on our pH-regulating systems. This is particularly true once we pass through our young-adult years. By our thirties, forties and fifties, excessive levels of stress within our lives can predispose us to chronic health problems triggered, in part, by overacidity. Practicing stress reduction techniques can help stress-prone people control their tendency toward overacidity and enable them to remain more healthfully alkaline.

Overly acidic individuals can benefit by finding a balance between the excitement and challenges of life and sufficient periods of rest and relaxation. Peaceful, calming activities such as meditation, yoga, listening to relaxing classical music, or taking quiet walks alone or with friends and family can help to promote a more alkaline pH within the body. In addition, taking frequent hot baths or saunas or even treating oneself to a massage periodically will have similar pH-normalizing benefits.

One easy way to alkalinize the body is by breathing slowly and deeply. The practice of yoga and meditation promotes deep, slow breathing. Deep inhalation oxygenates the tissues, while deep exhalation helps to remove carbon dioxide from the body. Deep breathing also promotes relaxation of the muscles and blood vessels. In addition, the normal outpouring of stress chemicals caused by the fight-or-flight response can be interrupted. Taking a short holiday from worry and stress by calmly breathing deeply can facilitate the restoration of our buffering capability.

Another way to promote the removal of acidic waste products from the body is by warming the interior tissues with hot baths, saunas, and massage. Once the internal temperature of the body is raised, the small blood vessels dilate, and circulation throughout the body is improved. An alkalinizing bath can be particularly beneficial for conditions such as stiffness and muscle tension, both of which are worsened by the accumulation of acids within the body.

To take an alkalinizing bath, run a tub of hot water, add one cup of bicarbonate of soda, and soak for twenty minutes. You will feel very relaxed and sleepy after this bath, so it is best to enjoy it at night before going to sleep. You will probably wake up feeling refreshed and energized the following day. Many harried and busy people have also learned that a weekly professional massage can greatly help to reduce their level of stress and thereby help to normalize the pH of the body. The areas of the body where a person is massaged are warmed as blood circulation is stimulated. This enables stored acids to enter the circulation and be eliminated.

Diet and Lifestyle Tips for High-Alkaline Producers

The following tips will help naturally high alkaline individuals maintain their tremendous physical energy, stamina, and resistance to disease.

Eat a Highly Acidic and Nutrient-Rich Diet

Naturally alkaline people are the only ones who can thrive on the dozens of acidic foods that make up the backbone of the standard American diet. Their alkaline mineral reserves and their production of alkaline buffers like bicarbonate are so great that a nutrient-rich, highly acidic diet will help them stay in balance and allow them to maintain their ability to perform at peak levels and remain in excellent health for decades longer than most other people, provided that their other chemical functions remain intact.

These individuals should emphasize nutritious foods that are higher in acid content. Unless they have a particular food sensitivity, they can eat all of the following highly acidic fruits and their juices: citrus fruits, berries, apples, apricots, grapes, pineapples, and tomatoes. Not only are these fruits acidic, but they are rich sources of important nutrients like vitamin C, bioflavonoids, and potassium. Most vegetables tend to be either moderately or low acid in their content.

Alkaline individuals can enjoy and even thrive on beans and peas, asparagus, artichoke, eggplant, lettuce, cabbage, broccoli, and many other highly nutritious vegetables. They can also benefit by dressing or marinating vegetables in vinegar. This popular condiment has a beneficial acidifying effect since it lowers the pH of the vegetables. Antipasti, cured olives, dill and sweet pickles, marinated bean salads, coleslaw, potato salads, and green salads are all normally flavored with vinegar-based dressings. In contrast, overly acidic people may find that the use of vinegar can produce heartburn, abdominal discomfort, and other acid-related symptoms.

Naturally alkaline individuals will feel their best on an acidic, meat-based diet. They tend to need several servings of meat per day. They can enjoy range-fed beef, lamb, and veal, as well as game meat, which contains a much lower content of saturated fat than most meat found in supermarkets. They can also benefit from omega-3 rich fish and free-range poultry. While fish and poultry are neutral to slightly alkaline when first eaten, their high protein content requires significant amounts of hydrochloric-acid production within the stomach—and results in significant amounts of acid-breakdown products.

Fish, poultry, and organically raised red meat should be chosen over the cuts of red meat found in most supermarkets, which are typically very high in saturated fat. The higher polyunsaturated fat content of fish, poultry, and organically raised red-meat products will help to protect naturally alkaline individuals from the heart attacks and strokes that they are prone to. In addition the total fat content of organically raised animals is usually lower than that of animals raised by conventional methods.

This does not mean that these individuals should eat the standard American diet with its high saturated-fat and refined-sugar content as well as its notoriously low nutrient content. Like the rest of the population, naturally alkaline people should avoid fatty cuts of red meat, dairy products, rich, sugary desserts, and the overconsumption of caffeinated beverages, alcohol, and soft drinks. Overconsumption of these foods will increase the risk of heart attacks, strokes, adult-onset diabetes, arthritis, and cancer of the prostate, colon, and breast as well as other common diseases even in these inherently strong and sturdy individuals. At the same time, these individuals should ignore the current belief that vegetarian-based diets should be eaten by everyone to insure optimal health. An exclusively vegetarian-based diet will make these individuals feel tired, edgy, and enervated. People with naturally alkaline constitutions are at their best eating a high-protein diet with two to three servings of meat per day.

Use Acidifying Therapies

A variety of nutrients and medications not only have beneficial therapeutic effects, but they are also highly acidic. As a result, these substances can be used to great benefit by naturally alkaline individuals. Several examples of commonly used acidic substances include vitamin C (ascorbic acid), acidic forms of calcium, and aspirin (acetylsalicylic acid). Other standard over-the-counter drugs like cough syrups and expectorants, which are usually manufactured as highly acidic, sweet-tasting products, are also better tolerated by high-alkaline producers or younger individuals with healthy buffering.

Naturally alkaline individuals should avoid the buffered forms of these substances, as well as other substances used to treat various health problems. They should take ascorbic acid instead of buffered vitamin C, calcium citrate instead of the more alkaline calcium carbonate, and regular aspirin instead of the buffered form. Thus, it is important to read labels and buy the proper acidifying substances and medications whenever possible.

Participate in Vigorous Physical Activities

High-alkaline producers tend to be drawn to strenuous types of exercise that are more likely to deplete both the oxygen content and the natural buffering agents contained within the muscles as well as to generate lactic acid. Physical activities such as jogging, weight lifting, competing in triathlons, competitive cycling, and mountain climbing will generate the acid waste products that help to maintain the pH balance of high-alkaline producers. These individuals also tend to do very well in rigorous team sports such as football, rugby, ice hockey, soccer, and basketball.

Many naturally alkaline people can maintain this level of intense physical activity well into their later years, provided that their other chemical functions remain reasonably intact. It is not unusual to see vigorous and naturally alkaline oldsters participating in triathlons and doing bodybuilding and long-distance swimming well into their eighties and nineties. Many of these individuals will also play golf frequently in their older years, populating the ranks of the many senior golf tournaments that are enjoying popularity all over the country. Walking a five-mile golf course several times a week is tremendously healthful for these vital seniors.

Lead an Active Life

High-alkaline producers thrive on fast-paced, busy schedules. They prefer to pack their social and business calendars with many activities. They do not tend to participate in the more alkalinizing pastimes such as meditation and yoga, which tend to be quieter and more contemplative. High-alkaline producers also tend to avoid low-stress, undemanding jobs. They prefer work and social activities that provide the level of excitement and even stress needed to generate sufficient acid within the body to counter their naturally alkaline constitutions.

Like everyone else, they do enjoy having time away from work and responsibilities. However, high-alkaline producers are never away from the action for very long since they thrive on excitement and stress. Their idea of leisure is to attend a boisterous boxing match or to go white-water rafting. While these types certainly do attend ballets and operas, they are often happier doing action-based activities. They may also prefer to listen to a heated debate or an emotional inspirational lecture rather than a dry academic class. Whatever activities they choose to participate in, high-alkaline producers will maintain a higher degree of physical and mental health if they remain busy and actively engaged in every aspect of their life.

Summary of Treatment Options for Restoring Your Acid-Alkaline Balance

A. Overly Acidic Individuals

- The alkaline power diet

- Restore your alkaline mineral reserves through sufficient intake of calcium, magnesium, potassium, and other alkaline minerals

- Use alkalinizing agents and therapies for quick symptom relief
  Sodium and potassium bicarbonate
  Sodium and potassium citrate
  Sodium phosphate
  Acid Check
  Buffered vitamin C
  Alkaline water
  Magnets
  Oxygen therapies

- Alkaline-enhancing habits
  Moderate aerobic exercise
  Stress management techniques like meditation and yoga

B. High-Alkaline Producers

- Diet: more acidic and nutrient-rich foods

- Better tolerance of acidic minerals like phosphorus and sulfur

- Use acidifying agents and therapies
    - Vitamin C (ascorbic acid)
    - Acidic nutritional supplements like hydrochloric acid and cider vinegar
    - Aspirin and other acid-forming drugs

- Acid-enhancing habits
    - Vigorous physical activities
    - Active, fast-paced life

www.ingramcontent.com/pod-product-compliance
Lightning Source LLC
Chambersburg PA
CBHW081101290526
45795CB00006B/1944